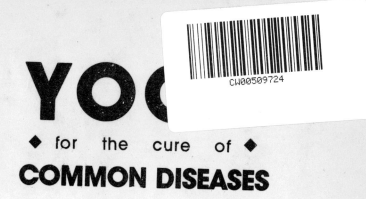

YO

◆ for the cure of ◆
COMMON DISEASES

Dr. Lakshminarain Sharma

Hind Pocket Books

©Hind Pocket Books,
1987 Edition

Published by
Hind Pocket Books (P) Ltd.
G. T. Road, Delhi-110032
Photoset and Printed at I.B.C. Press
G. T. Road, Delhi-110032

YOGA

◆ for   the   cure   of ◆

COMMON DISEASES

Contents

for an asthma patient: breakfast, lunch, dinner; use of medicines during attack; tried medicines. *Heart Attack:* causes, treatment, exercise programme, *Tanasan,* cycling, other asans, *Paschimottanasan, Shavasan,* diet regulations for heart patients, beneficial foods. *High Blood Pressure:* What is blood pressure, signs of high blood pressure, treatment, yogasan practice. **The Third Storey:** *Yogasans for digestive disorders: Pawan Muktasan; Yog mudra;* home remedies; natural treatment — mud bandage; liquid diet for digestive disorders. *Diarrhoea:* diet. *Dysentery:* home remedies, diet. *Diabetes:* Yogasan order, *Dhanurasan, Nabhiasan,* diet regulations; home remedies. *Jaundice:* treatment by food, other beneficial foods, treatment, beneficial yogasans. *Rash or allergy. Sunstroke:* treatment, precautions, some doubts and clarifications.

Preface

What is treatment? Treatment implies all those methods that help a patient to get rid of his disease and make him healthy. Eating the right kind of food, healthy living habits, nursing and administration of medicines are all included in treatment.

The modern trend is to turn to medicines the moment one falls ill. This is true not only of patients but also of doctors, Hakims and Vaids. Very little attention is paid to the other aspects of treatment. To clarify my point, I cannot resist the temptation of relating an incident that occurred while I was a guest at a friend's house. One day, as my friend was leaving for the market, his wife handed him a list of her requirements. The list included ten packets of a popular brand of pain killing pills, a bottle of antacid pills, and a box of purgatives.

"Why these medicines? and in such a large quantity?" I asked my friend.

"What can we do?" he expressed his helplessness. "My wife has to take one or two pills every day for her headache, otherwise she cannot do anything. I keep getting a stomachache. If I take these antacid pills, I feel better."

Obviously, these days people are getting used to medicines, whereas to be healthy, one does not need any medicines. What is needed is healthy living and the right kind of food.

The consumption of allopathic medicines is on the increase because they seem to give immediate results. Very few people are aware of the harm being done to them not only by medicines that are advertised extensively through radio, television, newspapers and magazines, but also in some cases by medicines prescribed by doctors.

On January 4, 1977, the Indian Science Congress held a seminar at Bhubaneshwar. Professor M. R. Das Gupta of the Calcutta National Medical College, said that because of the dangers of modern drugs, the medical profession itself had become a curse. He disclosed the reactions and ill-effects of different drugs. According to Dr. Das Gupta, many of the drugs consumed in the form of pills gave rise to after-effects that usually led to vomiting and haemorrhage of the stomach. Over-consumption of aspirin has increased the cases of bleeding from darts of the stomach. Readers must note that no pain-killing pill is manufactured without aspirin.

Tetracycline damages teeth. Antacid pills cause constipation and diarrhoea. Since all medicines that act within the body have to travel through the liver, the body cannot escape the ill-effects of the medicines. Prominent among such medicines are Phenaectin, Paracetamol, A.P.C., Sulfa drugs, Quinine, artificial Vitamin K and Tetracycline.

In fact, many modern medicines are responsible for heart diseases. Unfortunately, the number of such medicines is on the increase. Digiteline and Pronestyl cause heart disorders as their reaction sets in.

The side-effects of medicines like these are sometimes even responsible for heart attacks. Medicines that bring down high blood pressure, for example, block the nose. Amitryn, which is prescribed for dysentery, makes the heart weak.

8

There have been many instances of heart attacks and high blood pressure being caused by the use of some contraceptive pills.

The doctors themselves are now afraid of the side-effects of Penicillin. The examples given above are just a sample from Dr. Das Gupta's paper, which disclosed wide-ranging ill-effects of innumerable drugs. He even states that some medicines could well be the cause of cancer.

In fact, Dr. Das Gupta is not the first person to identify and call attention to the ill-effects of modern drugs. Many other media have also done so.

The April 1974 Drug Special of the World Health Organisation's journal, "World Health," is full of warnings about the ill-effects of drugs. Dr. B. W. Royal of the Drug Evaluating and Monitoring Unit, writes:

"There are thousands of drugs in the market today. These have a variety of ill-effects, like insomnia, vomiting, serious kinds of jaundice. These can cause disorders in the blood, and even cause death. Even a child in the womb can be affected."

By the end of 1973, W.H.O. had received over 75,000 complaints regarding the ill-effects of some modern drugs. These complaints refer to over 6,000 prevalent drugs. By now, it is certain that lakhs of more complaints must have been received.

According to the London "Times", there was a woman whose gums used to bleed. She was a healthy woman. She went to a doctor, who prescribed Chorophemicol, an antibiotic. After six weeks, she developed a cough. He gave her the same drug. As a result, she developed pimples on the face, her face became red, and hair began to grow on her face. She had to shave her face every day, her muscles also became like those of men. She filed a law-suit against her doctor. The verdict of the court was that such a strong drug should not have been prescribed for such a minor ailment. The doctor was asked to pay her 3,44,046 dollars!

The real question to be asked is, whose fault was it? The doctor's or the drug manufacturing company's? The answer to this is not simple.

Drug manufacturing has now developed into a very large industry the world over. Millions and trillions of rupees have been invested in it. Also this industry is an organised body. It has its own laboratories, its own chemists and analysts. Their main aim is to prepare drugs that will relieve pain at once (or at the earliest). It does not seem to matter how serious their reactions and after-effects are.

Their publicity departments are highly organised. They advertise through radio, television, newspapers, magazines, and large hoardings. Each company sends trained representatives to doctors.

Before World War II, when a patient went to a doctor, he would examine the person carefully. After much thought he would prescribe a mixture, and the patient was given detailed instructions that covered his food and living habits.

But today the situation has changed. In the words of W.H.O.'s Dr. Lloyd Christopher and Professor James Crooks of Dundee University, United Kingdom: "In today's age, a good doctor or a specialist, by and large, does not have the time to study the developments in the area of drugs and their effects. Representatives and agents of the various manufacturing companies are the doctors' sole source of information about new drugs. These agents only attempt to sell the drugs. They hardly ever indicate the ill-effects of their drugs. In fact, they speak fluent English to impress the doctors, leave coloured publicity material on their tables, and present them with free samples. The impressed doctor prescribes these new drugs, as if thereby he was fulfilling his duty. He does not feel the need to go deeply into the symptoms and case-history of the patient. To write a prescription after careful thought and consideration is indeed a thing of the past "

10

In fact, the drug industry appears to be buying the hearts and brains of the doctors the world over.

In this context, it is interesting to note that a pill that costs two paise to manufacture is sold for 25 or 30 paise. The costs, the commission of the agents and other expenses are recovered from the consumer.

EXCESSIVE USE OF DRUGS

The use of drugs is on the increase and this has become a problem. According to a poll conducted by W.H.O., the number of prescriptions is on the increase daily, running into lakhs. The more developed countries are consuming more drugs. There are other reasons for this, besides publicity.

In today's jet age, the ordinary man wants to get rid of his headache, stomachache or fever at the earliest possible moment. As a result, he turns to a "magic" pill. He does not even think it necessary to consult a doctor any longer. Either he sends for a drug that the admen have already sold to him or a friend suggests a particular drug. The habit of suggesting and prescribing pills for others' ills is an international hobby today. You have just to mention your ailment and you are sure to be flooded by sure-fire cures, grandmother's remedies and personal prescriptions. Self-medication can become in time a dangerous habit. The editor of the W.H.O. journal has written that not only should the common man be warned about the dangers of over-medication, but that he should also be warned equally against unnecessary self-medication.

Today one can buy pain-killing drugs, purgatives, laxatives and antacid pills from grocery stores, betel-nut and betel-leaf sellers and sometimes even from restaurants. People even consume capsules like Chloromycetin without seeing a doctor if they have a fever. A lot of people consume tranquillisers and sleeping pills without even a moment's hesitation. Doctors come across such cases of self-medication every day. Newspapers also publish reports

11

of accidents resulting from self-medication.

There are many groups of modern drugs. For example, Sulfa drugs, Antibiotics, Chemotherapeutic drugs, Cortisones, tranquillisers, etc. All these drugs can be extremely dangerous beyond a limit; therefore, the packing always carries a stipulation that these are to be sold against a doctor's prescription only. The accompanying leaflets carry a warning about the ill-effects of these medicines. A very clear warning is often printed regarding the consumption of these drugs without a doctor's prescription.

How dangerous it actually is to indulge in self-medication is a matter deserving deep thought. People who have the maniacal habit of prescribing drugs as a hobby should be particularly careful. An acquaintance of mine has this bad habit. If anyone so much as sneezes, he starts prescribing drugs! He is very enamoured of modern drugs, therefore he invariably prescribes the latest fast-acting drugs. He sometimes even buys the drugs and takes a promise that they will be consumed. He always carries a box of drugs in his bag and keeps popping pills in his mouth. Such people are truly dangerous, both for themselves and for others.

There are some who declare that the drugs prescribed by the doctor are wrong and those prescribed by themselves are the correct ones. Such people are even more dangerous.

However it becomes clear and certain that the demand for and consumption of modern medicines is on the increase. If we look into it closely, the reason for this increased consumption is basically the modern drug itself. These drugs do not cure. They only suppress the symptoms. The symptoms disappear, and the vitality of the body is reduced. The poison of the suppressed ailments remains in the body. After some time, these poisons may cause diseases like coughs, liver afflictions, gas and other digestive disorders, kidney problems, skin diseases, high blood pressure, and the hardening and narrowing of veins and arteries.

The patient then starts taking drugs all over again. Those who use modern drugs begin to depend more and more on them as time passes, until it becomes a vicious circle. Gandhiji very rightly said that once a medicine bottle enters a house, it remains there forever.

Dr. Kumar Swamy confirms this statement: "The tendency to give strong drugs to patients to cure them is on the increase. The ill-effect of this is that a medicine consumed as a cure, may well become the cause of a new disease."

A NOTEWORTHY ASPECT

I bought a cycle from a well-known company. The shopkeeper gave me a booklet along with the cycle. It contained certain suggestions for the buyer.

"If you want your cycle to give you good service for a long time, spend ten minutes looking after it every day."

It also explained how the cycle should be oiled, cleaned, how to drive it carefully, how to save it from rain and sun. Without doubt anyone who follows these instructions can keep his cycle in a fit condition and prolong its life. This applies not only to a cycle but also to every machine. Our body is a sort of machine, in fact, an extraordinary machine. There are some suggestions, some fundamental rules, that have to be followed to keep this "machine" in good shape over a prolonged period. If we look after our body daily for ten or fifteen minutes, we can enjoy a long, healthy life.

In fact, it is our own carelessness that makes us ill. Today many kinds of medical systems are available to us, like Homoeopathy, Allopathy, Ayurved, Naturopathy, Bio-chemicals, the Greek system, etc. All these have different fundamentals and principles. For example, the

13

allopaths believe that germs are the cause of any disease. The Ayurvedic practitioners believe that phlegm, bile and wind are the base for any treatment. Homoeopaths believe in destroying poison with the help of poison. Biochemists believe that there are twelve salts in the human body, the lack or increase of any of which causes disease.

But of all these systems, the principle of naturopathy is the simplest and most logical. It believes that the collection of useless or waste material in the body causes disease. The system holds that the beginning of a disease indicates that excessive poison has collected in the body, and it is time to flush out the system, otherwise it will become sick. Different kinds of bath, temperance in diet and fasts help nature in this cleansing process of the body.

But these days people take the help of naturopathy only when they are tired of drugs. If we were only to lead a natural life and follow the basic rules for good health, we would never fall ill, in the first place.

I have stressed the fact that prevention is better than cure in all my previous books. Some people follow the rules and remain healthy. But for various reasons, many people fail to follow them in a practical manner, and they often contract some disease or other. And then they feel the need for treatment.

Treatment is a technical job. Just as we send a machine to a mechanic for repairs, similarly the body also needs repairs. Yet there are universal rules that make the process of treatment easy and effective.

Immediate treatment is only required for a disease in a severe form, or for diseases that attack the body suddenly; for example, running a high temperature. In case of fever, the first step in treatment should be fasting. Even when afflicted by dysentery, diarrhoea, large boils, severe cough, vomiting, or severe pains in the stomach, one should stop eating. Drink a lot of water, so that the body poisons are washed out with urine. Clear the stomach. Mix

14

one kilo lukewarm water and juice of one lime and take an enema. Rest in bed.

With such simple precautions, the effect of a disease is minimised. Sometimes such simple treatments may even cure the patient. One does not then have to take any medicine at all.

THE AIM OF THIS BOOK

Like my other books, this book too aims to help you to remain in good health. Also I wish to impart scientific knowledge about treating common ailments at home, so that you do not have to spend unnecessary amounts of money on medicines and may save yourself the trouble of running after doctors.

As compared to my other works, this book is different. I have not followed any particular system, except perhaps the system of common sense. I have specially emphasised the yogasans and also incorporated instructions and rules about diet and general health. A special feature of this book is that I have also incorporated harmless beneficial medicines and effective home remedies. I have taken the same attitude while writing this book as I take while treating my patients. Because I am a naturopath, prominence has obviously been given to experiments tried under the system of naturopathy.

I am very concerned about the harm done by prescriptions that are passed on by hearsay or by those published in journals without adequate research. I am consequently very cautious about what I write. The prescriptions and home remedies described in this book are scientific, and I am convinced that there is no possibility of any harm coming to anyone using any of them.

Dr. Lakshminarain Sharma

15

Our Body: A Minaret

Our body is akin to a three-storeyed minaret, standing on two pillars called legs. For the sake of convenience, we shall start from the top and refer to the head as the first storey, the chest as the second and the stomach as the third storey.

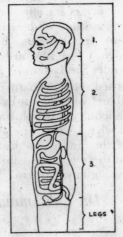

Fig. 1

THE FIRST STOREY

This includes not only the head, but also the parts above the shoulders — throat, face, eyes, nose, ears and brain.

To keep these parts disease-free, three yogasans are important. (1) Sinhasan (2) Udharvangasan (3) Matsyasan.

Sinhasan

Method: This asan can be performed either in a sitting or a standing position. To benefit fully from this asan, it is advisable to include Uddiyana Bandhasan also. Sit down with your knees bent, just as one sits for namaaz; place both hands on the knees, keep the arms straight; bend your body slightly forward from the waist, but keep your backbone straight. Do not let it coil or bend.

Take three or four deep breaths, then exhale completely. Pull the stomach in, open the mouth as much as possible, and stick the tongue out, open the eyes to the maximum and look straight — just like a tiger sticking out its tongue. (See Fig. 2).

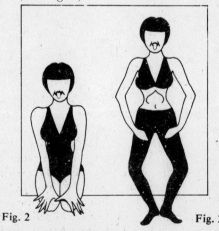

Fig. 2   Fig. 2a.

In this asan, the act of emptying the lungs by expiration and pulling the stomach inwards is Uddiyana Bandha. Remain in this position as long as you can hold it, that is, as long as you can keep the breath out easily. At the end of the asan, close your mouth, inhale and loosen all your muscles. Repeat after resting for a few seconds. It is enough to repeat this asan twice or thrice. In the beginning, you will be able to keep the breath out for a few seconds only, but gradually the period will increase automatically.

STANDING POSITION FOR THIS ASAN

The only difference is that you bend the legs slightly at the knees (See Fig. 2a). The rest of the method remains the same. You can adopt either method.

ADDITIONAL BENEFIT OF UDDIYANA BANDHA

Uddiyana Bandha has been included in the Sinhasan because it imparts good health by serving as a powerful gastro-intestinal tonic. A number of throat disorders start because of gastro-intestinal disorders.

Afflictions of throat

By and large, most people contract throat infections whenever there is a weather change. Cold, cough, irritation in the throat, and flu are all included in this. In this condition the membrane of the throat becomes swollen, and as a result of this, the throat becomes red. This swelling spreads to the nose membrane if it is accompanied by a cold, causing sneezing and a running nose. Although this is a very minor ailment, it makes one feel very listless. Some people may suffer for a long period, whereas others may recover within three or four days without any treatment for which a large number of medicines are available in any chemist's shop. A number of home remedies are also known. For the sake of truly good health, one should not suppress the disorder by consuming these

18

medicines. Try and understand nature. Nature wants to purify your body by throwing out phlegm and water from the throat and nose. Therefore, one should only take such treatments as make the work of nature easy and you will be relieved.

A large number of medicines for throat disorders are advertised through the media. The use of these only suppresses the symptoms, which in turn may cause other disturbances, like a headache or a dry cough. Often a disease suppressed by drugs reappears with greater force after a little while. Then people turn to more drugs to suppress these. I often come across patients who complain of frequent attacks of sore throat, accompanied by attacks of cold and flu. The root cause of this is the habit of drug consumption.

Never consume drugs under these circumstances. Instead the regular performance of Sinhasan proves very beneficial for all throat disorders. Those practising Sinhasan are never afflicted by any throat ailment. The throat muscles are toned up and as the flow of the blood reaches the diseased area, the ailment starts getting cured. While practising Sinhasan, you will soon find that heaviness and irritation are on the decrease. Phlegm becomes thicker and is soon completely gone, and tension in the inner portion of the throat also starts decreasing.

Sinhasan should be performed in the morning on an empty stomach. If necessary, it can be performed more than once in a day. Uddiyana Bandha need not be performed if Sinhasan is repeated during the day.

Remember the following:

Include Uddiyana Bandha only while performing Sinhasan four hours after a meal. Uddiyana Bandha can be performed along with Sinhasan in the evening only if one has passed a motion and the stomach has been cleared.

Sinhasan can be performed one hour after lunch (without Uddiyana Bandha).

19

It is not necessary to take the prescribed sitting or standing position if Sinhasan is being repeated. It can be performed while walking, in the lying down position, or simply while sitting. Once a Delhi lawyer woke up with a sore throat. He also experienced difficulty in talking. He had to argue in court that day. He was worried. He sent for a pill but it had no effect. He was familiar with Yogasans. He performed the Sinhasan every ten minutes. In between he sipped warm water. After half an hour, he felt better and started preparations for the case. While going through the files, he did not forget to repeat the Sinhasan. He refrained from eating any food. This step is highly favoured in Naturopathy. By the time he reached the court, his throat and voice had cleared up and he was able to present his arguments properly.

I have a young neighbour who had been afflicted with a sore throat for a month. It was not so much the throat as his voice that was affected. He came to me after trying various remedies. I advised Sinhasan. Within two days, he was completely cured.

TONSILS

Tonsils are categorised under throat disorders. Normally they are the size of berries, are two in number, and are situated on the right and left sides of the throat.

Tonsils become enlarged due to throat disorders. Sometimes it becomes a chronic disorder. By and large, children are afflicted by this more often than adults. Mostly the doctors advise removal of tonsils by an operation. But this removal does not make the operated person free from throat disease.

In the naturopathic system, tonsils or any other throat disorder is primarily thought to be caused by digestive disorders. It is not possible to get rid of these ailments if one's digestive system is not first improved. Suggestions for improving the digestive system will follow later in this chapter. Sinhasan is very beneficial for tonsil disorders.

FALLING OF THE UVULA

Often the palate becomes inflamed. At the end of the palate, there is a small tail-like formation known as the uvula. When the palate is inflamed, the uvula also becomes inflamed and 'falls' down. Thus it becomes difficult to gulp water, food or even spit. Sinhasan cures this disorder very quickly as the basic principle remains the same. With the stretching of the mouth, the muscles inside the mouth are also stretched, the rate of blood flow increases and the inflammation starts decreasing, due to the consequent accelerated cleansing action of the blood. For all minor throat disorders, perform Sinhasan, it is always beneficial and inevitably curative. Never consume the so called quick-acting "magic" drugs.

SECONDARY TREATMENT

There are many approved home remedies in naturopathy that cure throat disorders. While practising this asan, the following treatment should be followed concurrently.

GARGLES — HOT AND COLD

Early in the morning take a glass of lukewarm water and add a pinch of salt. Take another glass full of cold water from an earthenware bowl. Do not add salt to this water. Gargle twice with warm water, once with cold water. Repeat ten to twenty times. Always begin with warm water and end with cold water. This is very beneficial for throat disorders.

FOMENTATION — HOT AND COLD

Take a piece of khadi cloth half a metre long and five centimetres wide, soak it in hot water, squeeze the water, place the cloth on the outer part of the throat for fomentation. Repeat two or three times. Keep another similar-sized cloth ready. Soak this one in very cold water. Squeeze off the water and wrap the cloth around the throat. Wrap a woollen scarf over this. Keep it wrapped for one hour. This wrapping will definitely help cure inflammation, sore throat, tonsils, hanging ovula, cold, cough and influenza. The wrapping can be done at any time, but it is most beneficial if it is done just before going to bed at night. In this case, if the wrapping is kept for the whole night, no harm will be done. This may be repeated twice or thrice in 24 hours.

DIET REGULATIONS AND RESTRICTIONS

During throat disorders, like any other disorders, it is necessary to pay careful attention to diet restrictions. If the disorder has caused fever, one should fast for a day or two. One should take a little warm water while fasting. Take four teaspoons of honey mixed in warm water every morning and evening. One must avoid all sour foods. I have suggested in my other health guides that one should drink a glass of water mixed with the juice of one lime every morning. Under certain circumstances, I have even suggested mixing of four spoons of honey with lime juice and water. In this case, however, one should avoid drinking lime water, and eating sour pickles, chutneys, curd and spices, as they aggravate inflammation.

All sweet fruits like bananas, papaya, sweet apples and chiku are beneficial. Sweet oranges are also beneficial but one should avoid sour oranges. Inflammation in the throat may cause a particular kind of dryness. Oranges and other pulpy fruits increase moisture and humidity. This helps to throw out phlegm. Some people are afraid to eat these fruits because their effect is cooling. But this fear is baseless. Before drinking fruit juice in winter, place the juice glass in a bowl of hot water for a while. This helps remove the cooling effect. One should particularly avoid watermelons during a throat disorder. Their effect is excessively cooling. Muskmelon is strongly recommended. Along with sour foodstuffs, one should avoid cold drinks like soda, buttermilk, sherbets, etc. Nor should one

22

drink iced water. Refrigerated water is equally harmful.

Carrots, tomatoes, radishes, spring onions, etc., are often eaten raw. This is most beneficial. But during a cough and cold, one should not eat raw tomatoes and radishes as tomatoes are sour and the effect of radish is cooling. But raw carrots, in this condition, are very beneficial. The fact is that if everyone were to eat one raw carrot a day, he would never suffer from any throat disorder. Raw carrots are rich in vitamin A and they help develop resistance to disease. Cooked greens like spinach, fenugreek leaves, bathua and cholai are also very beneficial. Radish leaves can also be cooked.

SOME COMMON HOME REMEDIES

People in every region and province have their own home remedies for colds and coughs.

Hot jalebi or hot gulab jamun is beneficial. Halwa cooked in pure ghee is beneficial.

Any sweet made out of dried milk, if eaten before retiring, is beneficial. Avoid drinking water after this.

Buttered toasts and tea help reduce throat irritations and colds.

Eat hot carrot halwa before retiring but avoid drinking water thereafter.

Mix 25 gms of wheat husk in 200 gms water and boil till the liquid is reduced to a half. Add a spoonful of sugar. If taken hot before going to bed, it helps cure cold and cough.

All these home remedies are based on one principle — the throat should be warmed and it should receive "grease". This helps remove inflammation and dryness from the throat. That is why these home remedies are helpful. The same principle is applicable to the use of roasted gram in many regions.

All the above-mentioned home remedies are scientifically expedient and can be followed. One can eat food if

23

there is no temperature. Ghee and milk can also be taken. Those not used to a daily rice diet should avoid rice during a cold and cough. The condition improves if one eats a little less than one's usual fill.

TEA

Tea is consumed on a very large scale and a lot of people feel that tea is beneficial for many disorders. It is often claimed that tea is beneficial during a cold and cough. This is not true. There is no harm if one takes a cup of tea in the morning and evening. But people who drink twenty to twenty-five cups of tea a day suffer from frequent throat disorders. The reason for this is that due to tea-drinking, the throat remains warm most of the time and, as a result, loses its power to tolerate cold. Consumption of cold drinks, buttermilk, sherbets, etc., also causes sore throat. Only those who take little or no tea benefit from tea during a throat disorder. It is more beneficial to drink tea with ten leaves of holy basil (*tulsi*) plant.

BETEL-LEAF

Betel-leaf is very popular in our country, and offering it to guests is an old tradition. It is a highly beneficial leaf from the medical point of view. A large number of medicines prepared for colds and coughs contain the juice of betel-leaves. Two spoons of warmed betel-leaf juice and one spoon of honey are very beneficial.

Betel-leaf with lime gives immense relief to the throat, and irritation is reduced. The catechu *(katha)* makes the betel doubly effective as it helps reduce the inflammation. It also helps cure a hoarse throat.

A PRECAUTION

A large variety of lozenges are sold for quick relief of throat disorders. Various pills are advertised extensively for headaches, too. Most people are misled and attracted by these advertisements. As a result, their sales are going up. But all headache pills contain aspirin which reduces the headache for a short while. The claim of the manufacturing companies that these pills cure colds and coughs is not true. These pills can only suppress the disease, which later may take another form. One should never take these pills. The home remedies given in this chapter are far better than the pills and can have no harmful after-effects at all

Boils in the mouth

Although boils in the mouth are very much like throat disorders in some ways, they belong to a different category and their treatment is also quite different.

The reason for boils in the mouth is stomach disorders, particularly constipation, which generate heat and acidity in the intestines. When this heat travels upwards the boils begin to appear in the mouth. In their aggravated condition, these become so painful sometimes, that it becomes difficult to eat or talk.

Although Sinhasan does not cure boils, this asan, if performed along with Uddiyana Bandha, helps to prevent this affliction. The Uddiyana Bandha also helps cure boils, and stops their reappearance. This asan also helps the digestive system. The intestines remain healthy, and that prevents one from becoming constipated, which is the root cause of boils.

In allopathy, normally, vitamin B complex and vitamin C are prescribed for boils. Allopaths believe that the lack of these vitamins causes the boils. Most doctors do not think of clearing the stomach. That is why vitamin pills and injections have little effect. Even if there is slight improvement, the cure is not permanent. The boils may reappear a few days later.

COMMON HOME REMEDIES FOR BOILS

Gargling with alum water.

Gargling with water boiled with mulberry leaves.

While there are many other home remedies, they do not remove the root cause of the affliction.

SUCCESSFUL TREATMENT

Mix lime juice in warm water and take an enema in case of boils in the mouth. The method of taking an enema is given in the appendix. As the enema clears the stomach, and the boils start receding, one should drink a glass of cold water mixed with the juice of one lime and four spoons of honey three times a day. If the body is in need of vitamin C, the lime provides it naturally and in adequate measure. Lime also helps remove heat and acidity from the stomach. Lime and honey make the intestines humid and help to end constipation. A mud bandage on the stomach is also very beneficial. This bandage should be applied three hours after a meal. If the mud bandage is applied twice a day, boils are cured very quickly. The method for application of a mud bandage is also given in the appendix.

DIET REGULATIONS

Do not eat anything sour and avoid pepper and spices. In fact, it is often not possible to eat spiced food if one has boils in the mouth. Sometimes it is not even possible to eat salted food. Eggs and meat are also harmful, one should have light simple food. Milk, buttermilk, curd and ghee can also be taken. Almost all fruits are permitted. In summer, mulberry and watermelon are very beneficial. One can even drink mulberry juice.

Dental Disorders

Dental disorders are on the increase these days. One comes across advertisements of new medicated toothpastes and powders for bleeding gums, bad odour, pain and pyorrhoea. The truth is that no toothpaste or powder is beneficial for dental disorders. These disorders remain despite such "treatments". Nor is there a special asan for dental disorders. Teeth can only be exercised by chewing or masticating, which is their prime function. The first point in this context is to chew your food properly. Food eaten like this is disgested quickly and digestive disorders are avoided. This also exercises the teeth. A better exercise for teeth is the chewing of a fibrous twig of the margosa tree (neem). While one chews the twig to turn it into a brush, the teeth benefit from the chewing action, while the juice of margosa twigs kills germs. The twigs of the acacia (keekar) tree also have similar qualities. Besides, this twig is also beneficial for throat disorders. A very simple, effective and cheap prescription that may be beneficial to readers is given below:

PRESCRIPTION

Soda-bi-carb
Calcium carbonate
Salt (ground very fine)

Mix all these and store in a clean bottle. Chew the margosa or acacia twig into a brush and then use it to clean the teeth with this powder. Not only will this clean teeth, it will also be beneficial for dental disorders as calcium, salt, vitamin D, and vitamin C are all necessary for healthy teeth.

The very construction of teeth is based on calcium. Milk and curds are both rich in calcium. But calcium is beneficial for the body only if the body gets vitamin D. The best source of vitamin D is oil extracted from fish. But in our country, there is no dearth of sunlight. One should oil the body and sit in the sun. Normally Indians do not suffer from lack of vitamin D. Lime, oranges, guavas and most of all myrobalan (aamla) are rich in vitamin C. Gums particularly need vitamin C, and this vitamin is also necessary for making the body strong enough to resist disease.

Those who suffer from bleeding gums, swollen gums and those who find their gums hurt while drinking cold water should eat fruits rich in vitamin C. Lime, oranges and

27

guavas are seasonal fruits. But now lime is available in almost all the seasons even though a little more expensive. Dry powder of myrobalan (aamla) is available in all seasons. It is good to have a spoonful of this powder with a glass of milk or water.

Disorders of face

When talking about the face, my concern is with cheeks. Normally, cheeks do not become diseased except for pimples, dryness, wrinkles, etc. As far as pimples are concerned, only the young get them.

We shall not go into the causes of pimples, for there are many theories, but no unanimous opinion on the subject. Here, however, are some facts.

Pimples are connected with pubescence.

Almost every young boy and girl gets pimples.

Constipation and a malfunctioning of the digestive system increase pimples.

Green vegetables and fruits help reduce pimples.

The much advertised creams, ointments, and other medicines do not cure pimples.

Improved diet along with wet cakes of clean mud do help cure pimples. These mud packs should be tied to cheeks before going to bed at night.

Two spoons of dried myrobalan powder taken with a glass of water or milk help cure pimples.

250 grams of raw carrot, if eaten daily in winter, help keep the skin beautiful and adequately oiled. The juice of one lime mixed with a glass of water also helps reduce pimples. Along with these precautions, the performance of Sinhasan is positively beneficial. The flow of blood to the face increases while performing Sinhasan, making the skin healthy. The cheeks become rounded as a result of this asan and the skin becomes alive and radiant. The performance of Sinhasan and Uddiyana Bandha makes the face healthy and glossy and lends lustre to the cheeks.

Sarvangasan

Sarvangasan is also called the "Reversed Pose" because in this asan the body is involved, while the other asans are performed in sitting and standing positions.

Li· down on a mat or blanket, rest in the deep relaxation posture for several moments.

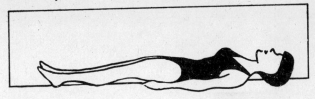

Fig. 3

Place your palms against the floor; tense your abdominal and leg muscles. Push palms against the floor and slowly raise your legs. The knees should be kept straight.

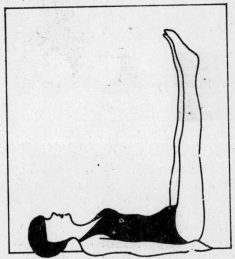

Fig. 3a

Swing your legs back over your head. As soon as your hips leave the floor, brace your hands against them to support your lower back.

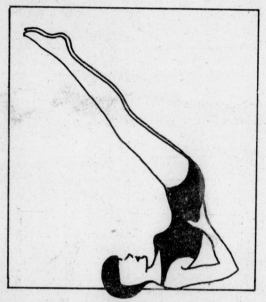

Fig. 3b

Very slowly and cautiously straighten to a moderate upright position. The legs should be relaxed, eyes closed. Bend your knees and lower them to your forehead. Place palms back on the floor and gracefully roll forward. When your hips touch the floor, straighten your legs into the position as in Fig. 3a, slowly lower legs to the floor and relax for one minute.

In the beginning, this asan should be performed only for half or one minute. Breathe only from the nostrils and to keep track of time, you may count. This asan can be performed for five to ten minutes. The duration should be increased gradually. The first two positions are for beginners only and can be deleted later on.

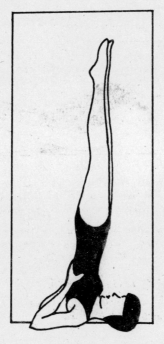

Fig. 3c

Matsyasan

Mastyasan is performed immediately after Sarvangasan. Spread a mat or a blanket and sit on it with the legs stretched. Bend the right leg and place the heel on the left hip-joint. Again bend the left leg and place the heel on the right hip-joint. This is Padmasan or the footlock. In this very position, lie on your back. The Padmasan should not be raised from the ground. Rest the elbows or hands on the ground.

Now lift the trunk and head. Rest the top of the head on the ground by bending the back well and throwing the neck well behind. Then catch hold of the toes. This is Mastyasan. If performed along with Sarvangasan, perform for two or three minutes only.

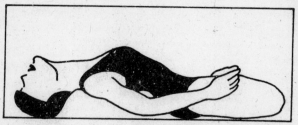

Fig. 4

It is possible that in the beginning you may not be able to perform footlock or Padmasan. In this case, you may simply bend the legs at the knees instead.

Benefits: This asan relieves cramps and stiffness in the neck, and common diseases of the first storey seldom trouble those practising these asans.

DISORDERS OF THE THROAT

During an attack of cold and cough, avoid Sarvangasan and Matsyasan and perform only Sinhasan.

TONSILS

Those suffering from enlarged tonsils should perform Sarvangasan and Matsyasan. These help the tonsils to become normal. Children above twelve years of age can also practise these. In case of a hanging uvula, both the asans should be practised along with Sinhasan.

None of these should be performed in case there are boils in the mouth. If, however, boils have just started appearing, it is beneficial to perform these three asans. By this method, along with the other treatments, the reappearance of these boils can be prevented.

DENTAL AND GUM DISORDERS

Sinhasan is not so helpful for both these disorders. Sarvangasan and Matsyasan are very beneficial. The diseased portions become healthy because Sarvangasan increases blood circulation. The poisons that have collected flow out with urine and perspiration.

DISORDERS OF FACE

Since Sarvangasan helps the thyroid glands to receive a good supply of blood, the skin and muscles of the face become strong. Pimples and dark circles under the eyes disappear. If proper attention is paid to diet and these three asans are practised regularly, the face becomes radiant and beautiful.

A SPECIAL BENEFIT

Due to the practice of Sarvangasan and Matsyasan, the thyroids and para-thyroids receive plenty of blood and are well exercised. Healthy thyroids imply a healthy functioning of the circulatory, respiratory and genito-urinary systems of the body. Thus these asans hold back the ravages of old age and keep you young. In most systems of exercise, the blood is made to circulate more quickly by means of increased activity. These asans, however, are an outstanding example of improved blood circulation without any excessive movement whatsoever.

BRAIN

Sarvangasan helps rejuvenate the whole system and improves power of concentration. The brain does not get tired easily, making it very beneficial for students. Nourishing food, however, is very important.

HAIR

Because these asans increase blood circulation to the brain and skin, they help the growth of hair, reduce dryness and make the hair soft and glossy. Besides ghee, milk and curds, you must eat raw vegetables and seasonal fruits. These are rich in salts, vitamins and minerals that are beneficial for the health and beauty of hair.

PRECAUTION

Never perform these two asans if suffering from high blood pressure, continuous headaches or permanent ear disorders.

Eye disorders

There are hundreds of eye disorders. Most of these are chronic like glaucoma and cataract. These chronic diseases may begin very slowly during young age, and if the treatment is not effective, may lead to loss of eyesight in advanced age.

A common disease that almost everyone suffers from is swollen eyes. The first signs of attack are indicated by a swelling in the eyes. The eyelids become red, accompanied by irritation. It becomes difficult to open one's eyes in the daylight, whereas darkness and coolness soothe them. Later, pus-like purulent matter starts collecting and flowing from the eyes. Due to this pus, the eyelids stick together.

Many home remedies are propounded, but it is doubtful whether these are scientific or even effective.

A large variety of ointments and eyedrops are available in drug stores. But these usually prove very expensive and take a long time to cure the disease. Sometimes they are ineffective.

One can contract this disorder any time in the year, but April, May and June are particularly bad. Common home remedies given below are inexpensive, easy to adopt, effective and scientific.

TREATMENT

Boil green Neem leaves in water, soak a cotton wool

34

pad in hot Neem water and foment the eyes. If this is repeated twice a day, the eyes will be cured in two or three days' time. If this does not give relief, take it that the eyes are swollen because of heat. In that case, do fomentation when the Neem water is cool. Make a mud cake and tie it to the eyes before retiring in the afternoon or at night. Within two or three days, the eyes will become normal.

FAVOURABLE TREATMENT

Constipation is responsible for this eye disorder to a great extent. Mix lime juice in warm water and take it as an enema. Early recovery is assured if the stomach is cleansed.

DIETARY RESTRICTIONS

One should not take rice, pickles, spices, pepper and curds as they are harmful for swollen eyes.

CHRONIC DISEASES

All chronic diseases affect eyesight adversely. The following methods can help check further deterioration and bring eyesight back to normal.

ASAN EXERCISE

Sinhasan and Sarvangasan are particularly beneficial. As the eyes, too, have to be stretched open during the Sinhasan, eye muscles are exercised. Through Sarvangasan pure blood reaches the eyes in good measure, thus making the eye muscles healthy.

EYE BATH

While bathing, our eyes are washed only externally. The inner parts remain unwashed. If eyes are bathed daily, they will remain healthy and normal. When we dive in a river, pond or pool, we are supposed to open and close our eyes under water. This is an eye bath. The following method should be followed in the absence of a river, pond or pool.

Method: Take a bucket or any other wide-mouthed container. Fill it to the top with water. (In winter you can take lukewarm water and cold water in summer). Immerse your face in the container, and keep blinking your eyelids and rolling your eye-balls.

With your face immersed in water, it is but natural that your nose will also be in water. So you will have to inhale and hold your breath as long as you can do so comfortably. To exhale, take your face out of the water. Repeat this three times at an interval of a few seconds. It is advisable to do this exercise just before your morning bath. This eye bath keeps the eyes clean and protected from many eye diseases, and helps cure eyesight disorders. One should not perform this exercise when one has a cold. Beginners may experience stiffness in the brain, but they soon recover from this feeling of discomfort.

HONEY AS MEDICINE

Honey is very beneficial if put in the eyes. If you feel your eyesight is becoming weak, apply honey to the eyes every morning and evening. The deterioration will definitely be arrested and your eyesight will revert to the normal gradually. A number of people have stopped using glasses by simply putting honey in their eyes. From the scientific point of view, honey is the nectar of flowers which gives strength to the eyelids and muscles. One can say that the eyes get food directly from honey. In the beginning, honey hurts the eyes and the eyes start to water. But as the eyes become cleaner, it hurts less Sufferers of glaucoma and cataract should use honey for a few months regularly and see the result.

It must be pointed out that it is very difficult to get pure honey. The commercially available honey is mostly sherbet of sugar or jaggery. Therefore, it is necessary to be careful at the time of buying honey for eyes.

THE SECOND STOREY

The second storey consists of the chest which has two important parts:

1. The Lungs — left and right lungs
2. The Heart — that circulates blood to the entire body.

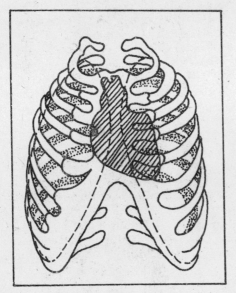

Fig. 5

The two lungs in our body perform a very important function for the body. Through the lungs we get oxygen which is the first requirement for remaining alive. We inhale and exhale in an uninterrupted manner twenty-four hours of the day and night. The importance of lungs can be judged from the fact that from the moment one is born till one dies, they are functioning continuously, without so much as a second's break. See Fig. 5a.

37

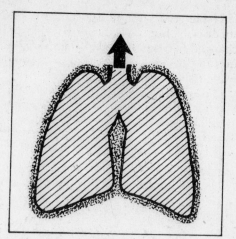

Fig. 5a

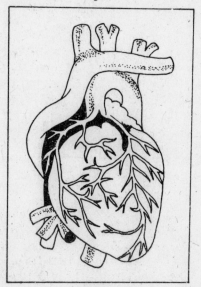

Fig. 5b

38

The lungs do not transport oxygen to the cells in the body directly, but cause carbon dioxide and oxygen to be exchanged between the inhaled air and the blood, which comes to the lungs for purification. When we exhale the used "dirty" air, carbon dioxide, is thrown out of the lungs and when we inhale, we take oxygen into the lungs where it is brought into contact with blood. The walls of the lungs have innumerable small holes which throw out and pull in the air. In this process of purification, nearly one-fourth of the body's blood is present in the lungs at any given time.

The lungs and the heart are the most important and delicate parts of the body. Perhaps that is the reason why nature has placed them safely within cage-like ribs that form our chest.

The following four Yogasans are beneficial:

1. Bhujangasan   2. Shalabhasan   3. Nabhiasan
4. Dhanurasan

Bhujangasan

Bhujangasan is a Sanskrit word which means a cobra. When this asan is fully done, it gives the appearance of a hooded cobra. The raised trunk, neck and head represent the hood.

Method: (1) Rest you forehead on the blanket or mat, keep arms at the sides, relax the body. Do not hold the muscles tight. Bring your hands up and place them beneath your shoulders. Slowly inhale and hold your breath.

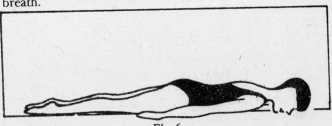

Fig. 6

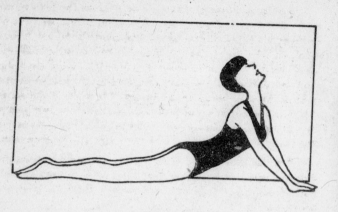

Fig. 6a

(2) In a very slow motion, begin to raise your head and bend it backwards. Bend your spine well. Do not raise the body suddenly. Rise gradually so that you can actually feel the flexing of the vertebrae, one by one, as the pressure travels downwards from the cervical, dorsal and lumbar regions and, lastly, to the sacral regions. Let the body, from the navel down to the toes, touch ground. In a very slow motion, reverse the movement while exhaling slowly, and lower your trunk until the forehead rests once again on the floor. Exhale completely. Pause a few moments before repeating. This asan can be repeated five or six times though beginners should practise it only twice for a few seconds each.

Shalabhasan

Shalabhasan means locust. When performed, this asan gives the appearance of a locust with its tail raised. This asan helps to develop, strengthen and impart good tone to the lower abdomen, groin, buttocks and arms.

Method: *First position:* Rest your chin on the mat with your arms by your side, palms on the floor.

40

Second position: Push against the floor with your hand and very slowly raise any one leg as high as possible. Keep the knee straight. Hold without motion for ten seconds. Lower the leg very slowly to the floor and raise the second leg in a similar manner for ten seconds.

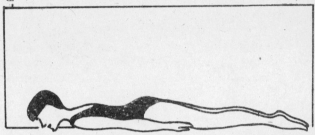

Fig. 7

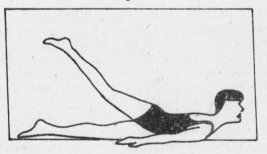

Fig. 7a

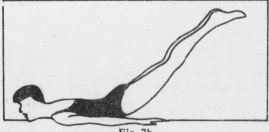

Fig. 7b

Third position: Inhale and retain breath. Push hard against the floor and raise both legs (one inch to begin with). The chin will remain on the mat, knees straight, breath held. Hold the raised position without motion for 5 seconds. Very slowly lower legs to the floor and simultaneously exhale. Relax for a few minutes. Inhale and repeat the asan.

Diseases of lungs

Introduction: There are many diseases of lungs. Mainly they are cough, asthma, tuberculosis of lungs, pneumonia and pleurisy. These are directly connected with lungs. Resistance to diseases of lungs increases in those who practise Yogasans. As a result, they are seldom struck down by these diseases. Bad health habits like smoking, drinking alcohol, and too much tea are responsible for these diseases.

A number of patients come to me with complaints of cough, phlegm, etc., and desire to be treated. But their history reveals that they are addicted to smoking and tea-drinking. In the beginning, they are asked to stop smoking and drinking tea. Those with a strong will power are able to control their habits, and their disease surprisingly starts getting cured without any medication. The pity is that those who drink too much tea are inevitably fond of smoking and alcohol too, bringing all the three 'fools' to roost together. So such a person, if afflicted with any of the diseases of lungs, must change these unhealthy habits. Those unable to control their habits may well suffer from asthma or T.B. at a later stage in life.

Once afflicted by pneumonia, tuberculosis or cough and fever, the question of practising yoga does not arise. Under these conditions, the treatment is quite different. Only those who do not smoke, drink too much tea or alcohol, and do not frequently run a temperature and have only cough and phlegm can practise yoga and expect to receive any benefit. Such people, before starting asans,

42

should go for an early morning walk for one week. They must go for a walk before sunrise and after morning ablutions. Later they should find a clean spot and sit down straight with legs folded over. Slowly inhale through the nose, hold the breath for a couple of seconds, and then exhale from the nose. Keep the stomach muscles pulled in. Perform the inhaling-exhaling exercise for five minutes to begin with, increasing the duration to ten minutes gradually. This is an easy Pranayam exercise. Special Pranayam exercises are slightly more difficult and a little more complicated. There is no need to go into the details of these here. This deep breathing is as beneficial as any good medicine. Blood is purified, the lungs are exercised and become stronger and the disease gradually disappears. As already indicated, after a week of morning walks, the practice of Bhujangasan and Shalabhasan should be started.

SUBSIDIARY TREATMENT

Wrapping and fomentation by wrapping. Take a khadi cloth or a towel large enough to go round your chest. Put it in a bucket or pan of hot water. Remove your clothes, take the squeezed towel, wrap it around the chest and sit or lie down. When the towel becomes cold, soak it again in the hot water, squeeze it and again wrap it. Repeat it once more. Keep a mulmul or voile cloth ready. Put it in very cold water, squeeze it and wrap it around the chest. Wrap a small shawl over it, secure it with a couple of safety pins. Keep it on for one hour after which you can dress. This can be repeated twice in 24 hours at any time except an hour before a meal or two hours after a meal.

EFFECT

This treatment helps widen the pores of the lungs and phlegm comes out easily. In summer fomentation can be done with cold water instead, but one must wrap a woollen shawl over the cold bandage. Keep the wrapper on for an

43

hour. This is beneficial for coughs, chronic or otherwise. It is also very beneficial for asthma patients. If taken on days when there is no asthmatic attack, and if taken every day, the attacks will become milder and less frequent. One can take this treatment during an attack too, but one has to be a little careful. The extent of benefit depends upon the temperament of the patient. First give hot fomentation a try. In case of discomfort, change to cold fomentation.

HOT FOOT-BATH

Take a bucket or a wide-mouthed vessel. Fill it up with hot water. Sit down on a stool and put both your legs in the water. Wrap a warm blanket or a thick cloth all around so that both your body and the bucket are covered.

Foot-baths can be taken for 15 to 30 minutes.

EFFECT

As you immerse your legs in hot water, the heat rises through to the entire body. As the warmth reaches the lungs, phlegm begins to flow and comes out easily. If the ribs are aching due to cold weather, the pain gets reduced as a result of foot-bath. If you are running a slight temperature, you can still take a foot-bath. The temperature falls as the body perspires. Keep the water hot by removing some of the water and adding more hot water, which should be kept ready. Hot foot-baths can be taken every day preferably at night for half an hour.

Once the body starts perspiring, the foot-bath should be stopped and the whole body should be dried with a clean dry towel. If the foot-bath is taken at night, it is advisable to go to bed immediately after drying the body. This induces deep sleep. If the bath is taken at daytime, do not go out for at least an hour.

PRECAUTION

During a foot-bath, if you feel heaviness or giddiness,

put a pad of thick cloth dipped in cold water on your head. Do not take foot-bath if this does not help. Those feeling discomfort during a foot-bath should not take it. But readers should not presume from this that a foot-bath is a dangerous treatment. One often feels heaviness or giddiness in case of a stomach disorder. In this case, one should take an enema to clean the stomach. There is no need for a hot foot-bath in summer.

HELPFUL HOME REMEDIES

The home remedies given below are tried, scientific, very inexpensive and easy to adopt.

(1) Mix half a spoon of ginger juice, half a spoon of basil leaf juice, one spoon of betel-leaf juice and four spoons of honey. Drink the mixture twice a day after warming it. Half or a quarter quantity is advised for children. Very beneficial for curing cough, cold, phlegm and fever. May be taken for asthma, too.

(2) Take clean linseed seeds and roast them on a tawa, grind them and store in a clean glass jar. Mix two pinches of linseed powder with honey and lick it three times a day. Half the quantity is advisable for children. Very beneficial for dry coughs and irritation of throat and sore throat as also for an asthmatic cough.

(3) Take lukewarm water (150 cc) and add four spoons of honey. Sip it slowly. Very beneficial for dry cough, fever and asthmatic cough. This can be taken three times a day. Half the quantity is advisable for children.

(4) Take thick cream from the milk pan, heat it, add glucose or misri. Eat it before going to bed at night. Helps cure dry cough, within a few days.

AYURVEDIC YOG-SITOPALADI POWDER

This powder can easily be prepared at home as all the ingredients are commonly available in the market.

Yog: One part cinnamon; two parts pipal (it is a

long pepper); four parts small cardamom seeds; eight parts vanshlochan (white earthy secretion formed in the hollow of a bamboo), 16 parts mishri. Grind all these very fine and strain through a thick cloth. Store in a clean glass jar.

Dosage: For an adult, 2 to 3 pinches mixed in honey. Half or a quarter of this for children. To be taken thrice a day (morning afternoon and evening).

If the cough is dry and the phlegm hard, add 2 rati (weight of one rati is equal to eight grains of rice) of sal ammoniac (Nosadar) to each dose. Very beneficial for hard phlegm and for patients of asthma.

A STRENGTH-GIVING YOG FOR CURING COUGH

Soak 10 almonds and peel them, wash 10 munakkas (dried grapes) and remove seeds. Take one grain of pipal, the ground seeds of small cardamoms (one pinch). Grind all these with a little water. Mix it with a spoon of honey and take every morning.

EFFECT

This concoction makes the stomach and throat moist and removes dryness which causes cough. Facilitates easy motions. Promotes hunger. A good appetiser. Almonds and munakkas are also strength-giving. This can be taken in winter, summer and the rainy season. Those suffering from asthma and frequent attacks of cough benefit from this. Give half or a quarter dose to children.

Asthma

Asthma is a very stubborn disease. There is a saying that asthma goes only when one dies. As an effect of the attacks, the pores of lungs become smaller, the muscles become stiff and the patient has difficulty in breathing and more than the normal amount of phelgm is formed. Constant coughing helps throw out a little bit of phlegm and the patient feels somewhat relieved.

There is no fixed time for an attack of asthma, nor is its duration fixed. It can last for minutes or hours or even days. The patient feels very weak during and after an attack, but after a while he becomes normal. Some people get the attack under certain circumstances as in a particular atmosphere. It may be aggravated by dust, heat, cold or a particular kind of food. It may even be caused by an odour. Mostly one has been found to be afflicted by this disease by the age of fifteen. This disease is more common in men. Women are less prone to its attack. Many a time this disease is hereditary.

TREATMENT

To date, no effective drug has been found for this disease. Drugs, particularly in allopathy, only suppress it. Most Ayurvedic medicines do the same. Out of these medicines, it has not yet been decided which one is really the most effective.

Different patients react differently to these medicines, as this is a very individualistic disease. The physiologists' quest for the cause of this disease is based on a variety of principles. Readers need not go into the complicated details thereof, but I would like to stress the root cause, and that is the stomach. The history of such patients reveals that they have often suffered from indigestion for a long time. Some patients get the attack when they are constipated. During an attack, the stomachs of some swell with wind. Therefore, the treatment of asthma should not be directed towards stopping the attack, but rather an attempt should be made to improve the digestive system by cleansing the stomach. Before talking about special treatments, I would like to draw the attention of readers to the fact that a patient should himself be aware and conscious about his own treatment. This proves very helpful. The patient should also be aware of all diet restrictions.

TREATMENT FOR IMPROVING DIGESTION

Drink a glass of cold water in summer, and warm water in winter mixed with four spoons of honey and one lime juice before morning ablutions. After ablutions, take a hip-bath, the method for which is given in the appendix. After the hip-bath perform the following asans: (1) Tanasan, (2) Paschimottanasan or Padhastasan (3) Pawanmuktasan (4) Bhujangasan (5) Shalabhasan (6) Sarvangasan (7) Matsyasan (those who practise Sinhasan may do Sinhasan) and (8) Shavasan.

For some reason, if you are unable to perform the asans, you can go for a brisk walk of a mile or a half after the hip-bath.

ENEMA

Enema should be administered once or twice a week when taking hip-baths, as it is necessary as an expedient to keep the stomach clean. The day an enema has to be administered, do not eat your breakfast. It should be administered an hour after the hip-bath and asans or morning walk. Just before it is administered, take a towel and dip it in hot water. Fomentation of the stomach with this towel for five minutes will help release the faeces sticking to the walls of the intestines and the stomach will be cleansed properly. The method for administering enema is given in the appendix.

MUD BANDAGE

Have an early dinner. After three hours just before going to bed, apply a mud bandage (the method for which is also given in the appendix). Repeat every day.

DIET FOR AN ASTHMA PATIENT

In the context of food, I want to emphasize that a patient is his own best friend. Anything that does not agree with the patient should be avoided. Since the roots of this

48

disease lie in the stomach, extra attention has to be paid to the digestive system. The patient should avoid straining his stomach. Follow the dietary instructions given below.

Drink a glass of water, or lime-honey mixed water before bowel movement. This is beneficial for lungs and faeces movement in the intestines. This is a substantial step towards improving digestion.

The morning bed-tea should be stopped completely, as it ruins the digestive system. Those changing their habit of taking bed-tea should not drink cold water. They should start with warm water.

Breakfast: If the patient is not too weak, he should miss breakfast, so that the digestive system can get a rest. But if the body is weak or if the patient feels too hungry, he can have a breakfast. Avoid bread, biscuits, sweets, namkeens or parathas, as they are very harmful for asthma patients. Use your common sense and understanding. If the seasonal fruit agree with the patient, he can have them. The best is porridge, cooked in water. A little milk can be added if it agrees with one, but never drink just milk for breakfast, as it is hard to digest.

Lunch: This meal varies from region to region. Those not used to a daily rice diet should avoid taking rice. Avoid lentils (dals), as they increase wind and are heavy on the stomach; marrow, torai, turnips, carrots, tomatoes, spinach, fenugreek leaves and bathua should be taken in plenty. If the patient is fat, avoid ghee. Curd should be taken only if it agrees with the patient, and does not aggravate his cough and phlegm.

Dinner: This should be similar to lunch. It is not beneficial to eat late and sleep immediately afterwards. It is advisable to eat dinner three hours before bed-time, particularly if a mud bandage is to be applied.

USE OF MEDICINES DURING ATTACK

Needless to say, an asthmatic attack is very troublesome for the patient. But there is hope that the frequency of attacks will decrease once the given treatment has been started and also that the duration of the attack will lessen. Unless the attack is severe, the patient should avoid drugs. Patients should instead take the help of the treatment described here. Drugs should be taken only if these treatments fail. I strongly advise patients to refrain from the use of drugs, because once the disease gets chronic, it becomes more and more difficult to cure. Drugs therefore should be used only as a last resort.

TRIED MEDICINES

For a long time, "Chitra Koot ki Kheer" has been famous as a medicine for patients of asthma. Every year in October on the day of the full moon, either a religious person or an organisation prepares a special Kheer (milk and rice pudding) one of the ingredients of which is a special medicine that is beneficial for asthma. A myth is prevalent that this Kheer cures asthma, as for a long time after, the patients do not get an attack. But as the effects of the medicine wear off, the patient sharts getting attacks again. Some do not benefit at all. There are some other well-known yogs besides this Kheer. But the claim that they cure is false. The main reason is that these prescriptions alone cannot remove the root-cause of the disease.

Heart attack

The heart is the second important organ in the chest. The function of the heart is to circulate blood to the various parts of the body. It is known as the king of the body because it fulfils such a big responsibility. There are many heart ailments, but heart attacks are relatively serious. In the last century, people were not familiar with this ailment, most doctors also did not know anything about it. Massive industrialisation and socio-economic development are largely responsible for making heart attacks very common. Heart attacks are today placed second on the list of killer diseases.

CAUSES

The causes of a heart attack are many, but the basic fact is that the normal functioning of the heart has been interrupted, resulting in a variety of heart diseases. I am only writing about heart attacks, because these are very common these days. Besides, the precautions advised for heart attacks automatically protect a person from other heart diseases as well.

A heart attack is a combination of myocardial infarction and angina pectoris. The heart supplies blood to the body but to fulfil its functions, it too needs blood. This function is performed by the coronary arteries. A particular kind of disorder in these arteries causes an interruption in the normal supply of blood. When the heart fails to get the required amount of blood, it fails to function normally. The main disorder of the coronary arteries is their hardening and shrinking. This is the direct result of unhealthy habits. Under these circumstances, fat starts collecting in the arteries. The fat contains a substance called cholesterol. Increased amounts of cholesterol may be caused by an unbalanced diet and may be related to the occurrence of atheroma. Later this may lead the patient to get a heart attack.

Arteries also supply blood to the muscular tissue of the heart. If they are obstructed or hardened, damage to the heart inevitably results. As the supply of blood decreases, so does the oxygen, because blood is the medium that carries oxygen. Under these circumstances, pain in the chest is caused for a short while. This is called angina pectoris. When the supply of blood stops for a longer period, then it is called myocardial infarction or heart attack.

TREATMENT

The question of using yogasans or home remedies during heart attack does not arise. Rest is absolutely necessary and the patient is often shifted to a hospital where specialists may look after him. This is the right step to take. Not all patients of angina pectoris or myocardial infarction die during the first attack; those of them who start yoga practice, follow strict dietary restrictions and take the advised precautions seldom get a second heart attack and can live a full and normal life.

Sports Medicine: Sports medicine is a new system that is gaining popularity and has been developed in European countries. After the treatment is over, and precautions to avoid recurrence are being followed, this system steps in. It comprises various exercises, games, gymnastics, jogging and hiking. This programme makes the body move. This system has proved to be more natural for the treatment, convalescence and maintenance of good health and is safe, inexpensive, easy and effective as compared to miracle drugs. It has given us a new viewpoint, and has changed the traditional lines of treatment. Writing about this change, Dr. Albert S. Heiman says, "I am attracted to sports medicine because it clears many doubts. Neither surgery nor medical science could clear these doubts."

I give two examples which indicate the changes taking place in the medical world as a result of sports medicine. Only one generation ago a patient of hernia, after an operation, was kept in the hospital for four weeks. If he was sent home earlier, it was considered as intemperance. Today if a patient is not sent home after two or three days, then this act is considered an intemperance.

After the birth of her first child, a mother had to stay in the maternity ward for ten days. Now they leave after two days. This system is based on the following basic principle: the heart should remain healthy and natural.

52

For this it needs movement. As long as the patient keeps lying in bed, the normal machinery of the body remains idle, and the chemical actions and reactions of the body stop functioning properly. Movement is absolutely necessary for a normal healthy life.

Today, medical science expects a patient who has suffered a heart attack to take bed-rest for at least six weeks. But sports medicine allows a little movement as soon as the pain in the chest is gone. In this context, the movement of legs is considered very important. Sports medicine considers a short walk the best exercise. The blood, it advises, should make one full circuit and return to the heart. This is only possible if the person has walked at least one thousand feet. There is no problem for outgoing blood but help is definitely needed for the blood to be circulated through the body tissues. Cycling is also a good exercise for heart patients. One can even lie down and move the legs as if one is cycling. Yogasans help heart patients to keep their blood circulation healthy and normal. Even heart specialists recommend asans today.

EXERCISE PROGRAMME

After recovering from a heart attack, the patient should base his exercise programme on the following rules.

1. Do not perform yogasans to start with. A short walk (1 to 2 kilometres) is advised for the first eight or 10 days.

2. After 10 days, start mock cycling (while lying down) and practise Tanasan.

Tanasan

Method: This asan can be performed in a sitting or standing position, but it is easier if performed lying down. Lie down on a mat or a durry, stretch the arms by your sides. Keep a little distance between the toes.

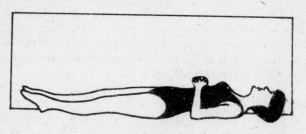

Fig. 8

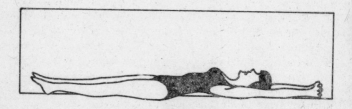

Fig. 8a

Remain in this position for about 15 seconds, so that
your breathing becomes normal. Bring both legs and toes
together, pull the toes a little forward. Place both hands
(with fingers entangled) on the stomach. Inhale and while
holding your breath, raise the entangled hands, with
stretched arms to the back of your head, place them on the
floor. Stretch your body. Slowly exhale, and at·the same
time bring the entangled hands forward and replace them
on the stomach. Return the hands to the original starting
position by your side and relax the body. Let your body go
limp and breathing become normal. Repeat the asan
twice. See Figs. 8 & 8a.

CYCLING

This is known as mock-cycling.

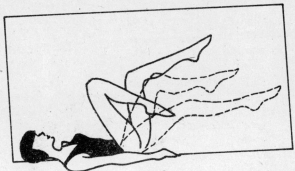

Fig. 9

Method: At the end of Tanasan, keep lying down face up. Move the legs as if cycling. This exercise should be performed quickly. Perform it for five minutes to begin with, increasing the duration gradually to 30 minutes. This exercise is to be performed twice a day.

OTHER ASANS

After Tanasan and cycling have been practised for a week, start the practice of the following asans.

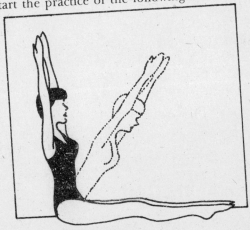

Fig. 10

55

Paschimottanasan

Lie flat on the back in a supine position on a mat or a carpet. Keep the legs and thighs fixed to the ground and stiffen your body. Inhale. Slowly raise the head and assume a sitting pose. Now exhale and bend yourself

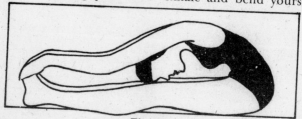

Fig. 10a

further forward till you are able to catch hold of your toes and can bury your face between the knees. Remain thus for 5 seconds. Slowly raise the body and resume the supine position. Inhale. Repeat the asan three or four times.

Shavasan

"Shav" means a dead body. When one performs this asan, it gives one's body the appearance of a dead body. This is the closing pose and must be performed after all the other asans have been performed.

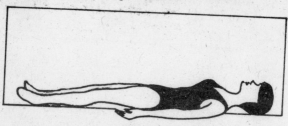

Fig. 11

Method: Spread a soft blanket and lie down on your back in a supine position, keep your hands on the ground by your sides. Let the legs be straight, heels together, toes separated. Relax the body muscles. Breathe slowly and rhythmically. Let your head lie on any side, relax, imagine that now you are tension-free. Imagine that a wave of relaxation is moving from your feet to the ankles, legs, thighs, hips, back, stomach, chest, arms, shoulders, and that it has reached your head (and brain). Remove all thoughts from your brain, do not think of anything, close your eyes and remain in this position like a dead body as long as you can. This pose is not only beneficial for heart patients but also for general mental and physical health. It gives a pleasant and exhilarating feeling. It is like recharging a battery. Inhale and exhale very slowly through the nose. You should not be able to feel that you are breathing. Do not make any breathing sound. As you perform this asan, you are receiving energy that is hidden in the atmosphere. In this pose, you will experience and enjoy perfect peace, ease, comfort and relaxation. It also increases your resistance to disease. Perform the above-mentioned asans in the following order:

Tanasan — mock cycling — Bhujangasan — Shalabhasan — Paschimottanasan — Sarvangasan — Matsyasan — Shavasan.

If you can afford the time, continue the morning walks along with asan practice. If you find it tiring, you can perform these only on alternate days. Those who use a cycle in the course of the day need not perform the mock-cycling exercise.

DIET REGULATIONS FOR HEART PATIENTS

Heart attacks are very closely related to food. Those who eat a rich, high-calory diet (particularly ghee and milk) and do not have to do much physical work, may ultimately suffer from heart disease. The work-load on the heart increases as the person habituated to rich food and no physical work becomes heavier and fatter. Those whose weight is more than normal should at once start reducing, even if they have never suffered a heart attack. There are two main methods, one is to do physical labour and improve diet habits. (1) stop eating potatoes, white sugar, rice and lentils. Stop eating fried foods, avoid meat and fish. Drinking of alcohol, cigarette-smoking and consumption of too much tea are an invitation to heart diseases. Alcohol makes you hungry and one tends to overeat. Nicotine, a poisonous substance in cigarettes, affects the heart adversely. Too much tea and coffee excites the heart unnecessarily and tires it. Doctors keep warning heart patients to refrain from all these.

BENEFICIAL FOODS

Research has revealed that raw onions, curd, butter-milk and black gram are very beneficial. Besides these, it is beneficial to eat all seasonal fruits and raw vegetables such as cucumber, carrots, tomatoes, radish, onions and half-boiled beetroots. These should be eaten in plenty. Avoid chapatis and increase the quantity of raw vegetables. This helps one reduce one's weight. If possible, do not sift the wheat flour used for making chapatis.

High blood pressure

High blood pressure is another gift of our developing age. The more developed and more affluent nations have a larger number of people suffering from high blood pressure. One adult out of twenty is afflicted by high blood pressure. More than sixty lakh people in America are permanent victims of this disease. The largest number of such patients are in Australia. The credit for ending the largest number of lives goes to high blood ressure. Modern medicine has not been able to give any definite or satisfactory reason for the cause of this ailment. Of course, much research has been done, much literature written and many theories have been offered. But naturopathy believes that bad health habits and diet are primarily responsible for this disease.

58

WHAT IS BLOOD PRESSURE?

The blood in the arteries is maintained under pressure. This pressure rises as the blood is forced onward by a heart-beat, and then falls as the blood glides along. Thus blood pressure is a measurement of both the maximum and minimum pressures of blood. One of two phases of the cardiac cycle is called systole. In this the ventricles contract to expel blood into the arteries. The second phase, when the heart rests is called diastole. There is very little pressure during diastole. When blood pressure is measured both systolic and diastolic pressures have to be measured. The normal systolic value for a young man is 120 and the diastolic value is 80. This will vary slightly in different people. It may also vary under different circumstances, depending upon physical or mental conditions. It becomes higher due to mental tension. Normally, it starts increasing with age. It also increases due to obesity. Excitement, hard labour, worry, fear and anger also affect blood pressure.

None of the modern drugs can cure high blood pressure. They only suppress it. No medicine can make the blood vessels elastic once the elasticity has been lost. Too rich food and lack of exercise make one lose this elasticity. The disease can only be cured if this elasticity is restored. Yogasans can definitely help. Elasticity can be restored to the blood vessels.

SIGNS OF HIGH BLOOD PRESSURE

The common symptoms of this disease are headaches, giddiness and tension around the eyes. In a prolonged case, the eyes can even be blinded or can start bleeding. Death can be caused by the bursting of a blood vessel in the brain. The patients tire very easily, some sweat frequently, the heart-beat quickens, and some feel an emptiness in the head.

This is a silent killer, often there are no other symptoms. Only if a person happens to go to a doctor for a check-up, is it detected.

Systolic	Diastolic	
180 mm	110 mm	High
210 mm	120 mm	Abnormally high
230 mm	130 mm	Serious
Higher than 230 mm	Higher than 130 mm	Dangerous

TREATMENT

Before advising Yogasans for high blood pressure patients, I should like to draw your attention to some basic health regulations.

Diet: Do not take any fried foods as they are hard to digest and only increase body-weight. As a result, high blood pressure may become chronic. Besides light simple food, raw vegetables and fruits are beneficial for patients of high blood pressure.

Medication: No medicine can cure this ailment permanently, so the use of drugs is useless. But amla is very beneficial. It has hidden substances that bring back elasticity to blood vessels. Fresh amlas are available in January, February and March and can be used in a variety of ways.

1. Make holes in amlas and extract juice. Mix a spoonful of ginger juice, two spoons of honey and four spoons of amla juice. Drink this mixture once a day.

2. Grind 2 amlas and 10 grams of ginger. Mix a little sugar and eat it every morning. Ginger gives energy and balances the cooling effect of amlas. Dried amlas can be used during the rest of the year.

During summer, soak 10 grams of amlas in half a cup of water. Crush the amla in the morning and strain through a muslin cloth or strainer. Mix in 2 spoons of honey and drink it. During the monsoon mix a spoonful of dried amla powder in a hot glass of milk and drink it at night. Dried amla does not suit some people. They may prefer amla murabba. But as murabba is less beneficial, do not take more than two such amlas in a day.

YOGASAN PRACTICE

High blood pressure patients should not practise difficult asans as this can be harmful. Begin with Tanasan and Shavasan. After one week, add mock cycling to the practice. Shavasan must always be performed at the end of every asan practice session. Shavasan relaxes the body and is very beneficial for high blood pressure patients. After three weeks, start performing Tanasan for three and mock cycling for 5 minutes. Pawan Muktasan, Paschimottanasan, Bhujangasan, Shalabhasan and Shavasan should also be started. These asans should be repeated according to your strength. In the fourth week include Sarvangasan and Matsyasan in the above-mentioned regimen of asans. Increase the duration of Sarvangasan gradually.

Stop drinking tea, coffee and alcohol completely. Smoking and tobacco-eating also increase blood pressure.

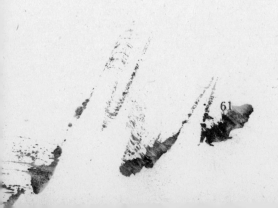

THE THIRD STOREY

The third storey of our body (stomach) is more complicated as compared to the first and second storeys. This is so because it houses more organs than the others: stomach, spleen, twenty-two feet of intestine, kidneys and the urinary bladder. The female reproductive glands, the womb and male seminal parts are also in this storey.

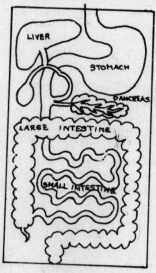

Fig. 12

Yogasans for digestive disorders

There are innumerable kinds of digestive disorders, but constipation is the most important, as most digestive disorders are caused by constipation. Enlarged liver and other allied disorders are also the result of constipation.

All the asans described earlier are beneficial for constipation, although the most effective is Pawan Mukt-asan. Perform the following asans in the order given:

1. Tanasan   2. Pawan Muktasan   3. Paschimottanasan
4. Sarpasan   5. Shalabhasan   6. Sinhasan and Uddiyana
Bandha 7. Matsyasan   8. Sarvangasan   9. Shavasan.

Pawan Muktasan

Lie down on a mat. Exhale and stop breathing. Lift left leg, bend it, bring it up to the stomach. Let the knee touch the chin with the rest of the leg touching the chest, press down on the leg, so that the stomach and chest receive pressure.

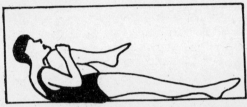

Fig. 13

Lift your neck and place your chin on the knee. Remain in this position as long as you can hold your breath. Then breathe slowly, and straighten your leg. Put your head back on the floor. Repeat with the right leg.

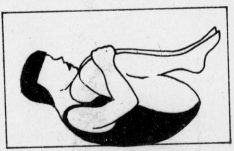

Fig. 13a

Repeat the same with both legs, as shown in Fig. 13a. Repeat three times.

Effect: Because the stomach is pressed and then allowed to go limp in this asan, the liver, urinary bladder, spleen, intestines and stomach are well exercised by it. Due to the practice of this asan, an enlarged liver will start returning to normal and the functioning of the liver will improve. It helps one get rid of constipation, improves appetite, releases wind and reduces gas.

Yoga Mudra

Sit on a blanket. Form a foot-lock (Padmasan) by placing the right foot over the left thigh and the left foot over the right thigh. Slowly bend forward and touch the ground with the forehead. Take your hands to the back and catch hold of the left wrist with the right hand. As you bend down, exhale slowly. Remain in this position for 10 seconds. Resume the original sitting posture and inhale slowly.

Repeat the Mudra three times.

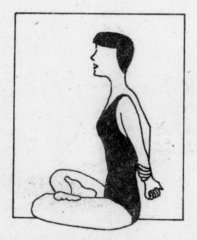

Fig. 14

64

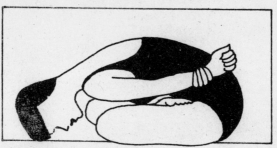

Fig. 14a

Improve upon the Mudra after a few days of practice, by drawing both feet up to the pelvic girdle with the heels against the lower abdomen. Changing of ankles puts pressure on the intestines.

Effect: Normally, the movement of the faeces in the intestines takes place naturally. In the constipated condition, however, this movement stops, and the faeces remain in the intestines. Yoga-Mudra helps to start this movement again.

Those suffering from frequent attacks of constipation should drink a glass of water immediately after passing urine and then practise Yoga-Mudra. It removes all disorders of the abdominal viscera. Those addicted to tea should start drinking a glass of warm water for bowel movement. Drinking plenty of water and going for a walk also help cure constipation.

HOME REMEDIES

1. Add salt and roasted and ground cumin seed (zeera) to thick buttermilk. Beneficial for enlarged liver, general functioning of liver and indigestion. (If you feel gas is formed by drinking thick buttermilk, then avoid it.)

2. Ten or 15 minutes before meal-time, eat a few slices of salted ginger. This improves the appetite and digestion and also reduces formation of gas in the stomach.

3. Mix one gram Sulemani salt in a glass of drinking water

and drink after meals. This cures liver disorders and is beneficial for the digestive system. It is also helpful in reducing gas.

4. Mix a pinch of soda bicarb with a pinch of ground omum seeds (ajwain). This aids the cure of stomachache, indigestion and swelling caused by overeating.

5. In winter, suck sugarcane on an empty stomach. This gives strength to the body, cures liver disorders, and increases urine output.

NATURAL TREATMENT: MUD BANDAGE

(See appendix for the method.)

If a mud bandage is applied for one or two hours, three hours after a meal, it helps cure a variety of digestive diseases, like liver disorders, constipation, loss of appetite, gas and acidity.

LIQUID DIET FOR DIGESTIVE DISORDERS

It is very beneficial to drink a glass of water, preferably mixed with the juice of one lime and a spoonful of honey. This is due to the fact that the intestines become dry due to constipation, which makes the faeces dry, and bowel movement becomes difficult. Water, lime and honey create lubrication and constipation is eased.

Constipation also causes acidity. The main signs of this are a burning sensation in the chest and the collection of a sour fluid in the mouth. Drinking water with lime and honey removes this disorder.

Most people have bread, rusks, biscuits, namkeen, sweets and tea for breakfast. These are very harmful for those suffering from indigestion. Fried foods made with white flour are very harmful for the liver, and promote digestive disorders. Those who eat an early lunch should avoid breakfast. They can have sprouted black gram (moong). The rest of the meal should be the same as advised for heart patients in the last chapter. Green leafy vegetables, seasonal raw vegetables and fruit should be included in meals. Chapatis made from wheat that has not been sifted are very beneficial for those suffering from constipation. The wheat husk is rough and it helps push out the faeces.

Diarrhoea

Diarrhoea is common in summer and is caused by heat in the stomach. Yogasans are not at all helpful for this condition. If you are practising Yogasans, do not perform them till loose motions have stopped. The following home remedies are beneficial:

1. Add lime juice and salt to water and sip it in small quantities.
2. Add half a teaspoon of Lavan Bhasker Chooran to 50 grams of curd. Drink it three times a day.
3. Take one kilo of clean, cold water, squeeze into it the juice of one lime. Take an enema. It is very beneficial.
4. Mud bandages applied twice or thrice to the stomach are very beneficial.
5. Take four or five ripe fig flowers (Goolar). Grind them. Add to curd, salt, black salt, roasted cumin seeds and roasted asafoetida. Fig flowers are only available in summer. Take once a day.
6. Clean dry pomegranate seeds. Grind them with a little water. Add a few mint leaves, salt and black salt. Grind it all into a chutney. Take 1/8th of a spoon five or six times a day. Very beneficial for curing loose motions during summer.

DIET

It is advisable to fast for one day. Drink lime water during the day. If it is not possible to fast, you can take orange or mausambi juice. You can also have khichari or rice and curd. Bananas are beneficial, too.

Dysentery

Dysentery usually starts abruptly with diarrhoea, lower abdominal cramps. The diarrhoeal stool is often mixed with blood and mucus. This is also a serious disease like diarrhoea. In this case, too, asans are not beneficial and should be stopped till totally cured.

HOME REMEDIES

1. Mix the pulp of a ripe wood apple (Bael) with curd and eat it two or three times a day.

2. Take 20 grams aniseed and soak in a cup full of water for one hour. Crush the aniseed and strain it through a muslin cloth. Eat two figs and drink the aniseed extract. This should be taken two or three times a day. Aniseed extract should be prepared fresh every time it is to be taken. If figs are not available, you can drink just the aniseed extract which itself is also very beneficial.

3. Take 25 grams aniseed and roast it. Add 25 grams unroasted aniseed and 25 grams dried ginger. Grind all three and mix with 75 grams of unrefined sugar. Store in a glass jar. Eat 10 grams three times a day with a glass of water. It is very beneficial for dysentery.

4. Mud bandages are also very beneficial.

5. Take an enema of one kilo luke-warm water mixed with the juice of one lime and eight spoons of honey.

6. Ten to 20 grams of Isabgol (a medicinal plant) mixed with curd should be taken two or three times a day. This is a very beneficial and popular home remedy.

DIET

It is very good to fast for one day. The same food restrictions are applicable to patients of dysentery as those given for diarrhoea. Diarrhoea patients should not eat green vegetables. If it is a chronic case, it is beneficial to drink the pulp of wood apple mixed with water and unrefined sugar and strained.

Diabetes

Diabetes is the excessive production of urine due to an inadequate supply of a hormone (insulin) secreted by the pancreas. Modern medicine controls it by giving an appropriate hormone to the patient. Insufficient insulin raises the blood sugar level. The urine, which may be copious, contains glucose. Consequently the patient becomes weak, and feels very hungry and thirsty.

There is no medicine in ayurved or in allopathy that can "cure" a diabetic patient. Through the regular practice of Yogasans, it can be completely cured, and insulin starts flowing normally again.

YOGASAN ORDER

Tanasan — Sarpasan — Shalabhasan — Pawan Muktasan — Dhanurasan — Paschimottanasan — Sarvangasan — Matsyasan — Uddiyana Bandha — (no need to perform Sinhasan) — Shavasan.

All these have been described in the preceding chapters except Dhanurasan.

Dhanurasan

When this asan is performed, it gives the appearance of a bow. Dhanur means a bow. The stretched hands and legs represent the string of a bow, the body and thighs represent the bow proper.

Lie prone on a blanket. Relax the muscles. Now bend the legs over the thighs. Firmly hold the right ankle with the right hand and the left ankle with the left hand. Raise the head, body and knees by tugging at the legs with the hands, so that the whole burden of the body rests on the abdomen and the spine is nicely arched backwards like a bow. Maintain the pose for a few seconds and then relax

69

the body. Even a weak person can perform this asan easily. To perform this asan, a sudden movement of the body is required. Be steady. Never jerk the body. This asan is a combination of Bhujangasan and Shalabhasan with the addition of catching the ankle. Shalabhasan, Dhanurasan, and Bhujangasan form a combination.

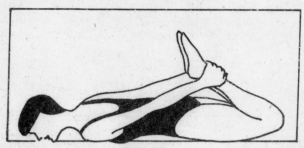

Fig. 15

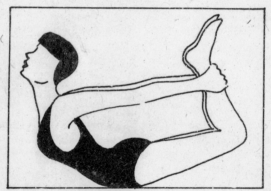

Fig. 15 a

These form one set of asans. Dhanurasan should be repeated 3 to 4 times.

Effect: All benefits of Shalabhasan and Bhujang-asan are derived from Dhanurasan. The back muscles get a

70

good massage, it helps remove constipation, cures gastro-intestinal disorders, energises digestion, invigorates appetite, relieves congestion of blood in abdominal viscera, insulin slowly begins to be formed and starts flowing out.

Dhanurasan is a difficult asan and many people cannot do it easily. Particularly those who are fat find it hard to master. Such people can alternately perform Nabhiasan.

Nabhiasan

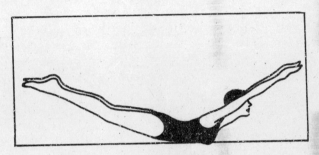

Fig. 16

Lie down on your stomach. Within a few seconds bring your breathing to normal. Stretch both arms in front of your head and bring both legs together. Inhale, and hold the breath. Stiffen the entire body and raise the arms, head, chest and legs simultaneously. The position should be such that only the navel and the area around it should touch the ground. Raise arms, legs and chest as much as possible. Hold the inhaled breath as long as you can and remain in the asan. Exhale and slowly bring the raised parts of the body down. Rest for a while. Repeat the asan three times.

Effect: The effect of this asan is the same as that of Dhanurasan.

71

DIET REGULATIONS

Special diet in which carbohydrates and sugar are restricted is advised for a diabetic patient, because he cannot digest a large intake of carbohydrates without the blood-sugar rising. The diabetic patient should avoid ghee, oils and rice. Most harmful is white sugar. Ripe wood-apple and other sweet fruits are beneficial. Two glasses of water with juice of two limes should be taken during the day.

HOME REMEDIES

A number of home remedies are common; some of the effective yogs are given below:

1. Take a few leaves of bitter gourd (karela) creeper, mix them with 10 grams of black pepper. Grind and drink it on an empty stomach every morning.

2. Take 7 leaves of black plum (jamun), 7 leaves of wood apple, 14 leaves of basil (tulsi) and 20 whole black pepper. Grind all these with very little water and roll the mixture. Make balls the size of small berries and dry in the shade. Store in a clean dry bottle. Eat one pill in the morning and another in the evening.

3. Soak one teaspoonful of fenugreek (methi) seeds in half a cup of water. Crush the seeds in the morning. Strain through thick cloth and drink it on an empty stomach.

Many other home remedies are popular in various regions. But one should not expect to be cured with the help of these. They help, but do not eradicate the disease. To be fully cured, Yogasans are beneficial because they activate the inner parts of the stomach.

Diabetes also falls in the category of chronic diseases. Therefore, it takes a long time to cure. Frequent urine tests during the treatment are helpful. A doctor's attention is also required. If possible, remain in touch with a reputed naturopath. The fact is that injected insulin has been proved to be an unsuccessful experiment. A number of experienced and honest doctors are now against insulin. Food, in this context, is very important. Raw vegetables and fruit are very beneficial.

Jaundice

Jaundice is a yellow discolouration of the skin and tissue due to the accumulation of bilirubin. There are three groups of causes. Liver disease, obstruction of bile ducts and haemolysis. The colour of the urine and perspiration (in an aggravated state) becomes yellow. The under-clothes as a result of the perspiration also become yellow. The body becomes weak, appetite decreases and the patient becomes constipated.

Modern medicine has no effective drug for curing jaundice. It is also considered a contagious disease (through water). The medicines administered for curing this are more harmful than helpful. These medicines, due to their strong reaction, aggravate the disease. In the case of jaundice, it is advisable to use medicines that have a cooling effect. A specialist has admitted to me that naturopathy can cure jaundice more quickly.

The most suitable treatment for this disease is correct food and health habits.

TREATMENT BY FOOD

If the attack is severe, it is better to fast for three to seven days. During fast, one can take fruit juice, pulpy fruits, and raw vegetables. Drink a lot of water. Bilious disorders of the blood are cured if fruit and vegetables are eaten. By increased drinking of water, the urine output is increased, which helps eradicate bile, unnecessary heat and other toxic substances from the body.

Depending on your strength, fast for as many days as you can. Then start eating boiled vegetables and chapati (without sifting the flour). Avoid ghee, potatoes, lady's fingers and egg plant. Green vegetables like marrow, ghia, tinda, parval and other green leafy vegetables like spinach, bathua, radish, and turnips are very beneficial.

OTHER BENEFICIAL FOODS

All fruits and fruit juices, particularly sugarcane juice, are very beneficial. Milk and buttermilk are also beneficial, but avoid cow's milk. All fried foods, ghee and oils are harmful and should be avoided.

TREATMENT

Soak 20 grams of roughly ground triphala (3 kinds of myrobalan) in 150 grams water in a glass or stone-bowl. Crush triphala in the morning and strain it. Mix it with ten grams of honey and drink it. Avoid this treatment in a severe winter.

BENEFICIAL YOGASANS

If the attack is severe, perform only Tanasan. It is advisable not to strain the liver. It is beneficial to take a walk bare-footed on the lawn. When the condition improves, start performing the following asans in the given order:

Tanasan — mock cycling — Pawan Muktasan — Paschi-mottanasan — Sarpasan — Shalabhasan — Shavasan.

Rash or allergy

This is an ailment that is connected with the liver. Red-coloured rash erupts on the skin as a result of heat created in the body due to liver disorders. Although a serious ailment, it does not last very long. But if it is ignored, if can become chronic.

Since the patient becomes very uncomfortable due to acute itching, there are many common home remedies. For example, people drink peppers mixed in ghee; red mud is rubbed on the body, which is then wrapped in a blanket. But these have no scientific basis and have no immediate or long-lasting effect. Modern medicine has many anti-allergic pills to offer. These days cortisons are being given which can control the ailment but also can do a lot of harm to the body. Beware of such drugs. The earliest, most harmless and most effective treatment for this ailment is fasting. Drink water mixed with lime juice and honey two or three times a day. On the second day of fasting, apply mud bandage on the stomach. Take an enema with warm water and lime juice. One can fast for three, four or five days. If no wheat or food is eaten for one week, the disease will be completely cured. If the disorder continues in spite of this treatment, drink fresh cool water into which are mixed two pinches of soda bicarb twice a day. Bile develops during this disorder, and the soda bicarb helps end it.

When cured by this treatment, eat pulpy fruits on the first day, boiled vegetables and fruit on the second day. One can start having chapatis (made with unsifted flour) and green leafy vegetables. A hip-bath for a week is very beneficial if the symptoms reappear. Hip-baths can be taken for one week. Psychologists are of opinion that fear, worry, distress, sorrow or grief causes this disorder. In these circumstances, it is better to avoid treatment of the body and consult a good psychologist.

Sunstroke

In summer, when hot winds blow, a lot of people become sick. There may be a feeling of listlessness, tiredness, fever and even fainting. The feeling of sickness is not caused by the hot winds, but a strong sun's rays. It just so happens that hot winds blow when the sun's rays are strongest. The same effect is created in hot places like coal-mines. The chances of contracting a sunstroke are great in places that are humid. Every year a large number of people suffer from sunstroke. Some even die of it. More cases of such sunstroke are reported in villages because the farmers work in the open. Strong sun's rays affect the brain.

Exposure to excessive heat results in prompt cardiac output and sweating. The salt content of sweat increases with rising temperature. Break-downs due to circulatory failure of the sweating mechanism are liable to take place. Cessation of sweating may indicate an impending stroke or collapse.

TREATMENT

The treatment is aimed at reducing temperature. Place the patient in a cool shady place and remove his clothing. Cool him by fanning after sprinkling water on his body.

Modern medicines advocate immersing the patient in cold water or using icepacks. We advocate ice-water enemas. Do not lower the rectal temperature below 39° C (102° F) too rapidly. Massage the extremities to maintain circulation. Sedatives are harmful.

PRECAUTIONS

Patients with a heat stroke should avoid immediate re-exposure to heat. Hyper-sensitivity to high temperature may remain for a considerable time. The patient should refrain from going out in heat or wear a cap or a hat or a pagadi if he must go out. Before setting out, drink plenty of water. See to it that the patient is not constipated, as there is great possibility of a further attack of heat stroke in case the stomach is not clear.

SOME DOUBTS AND CLARIFICATIONS

Most people believe that one can escape a heat stroke if one carries an onion in the pocket. This is not a scientific fact. Heat has no connection with an onion in the pocket. Also people think the pulp of roasted green mangoes with white cumin seeds, black salt and sugar (panna) is beneficial. This too is unscientific. One should never indulge in such prescriptions.

Diseases of Limbs

Legs and arms are branched portions of the body that are afflicted with specific disorders. The commonest are rheumatic disorders. Rheumatoid arthritis is a chronic disabling systemic inflammatory disease of an undetermined origin. It can involve not only the joints but also most tissues of the body, particularly the lymph nodes, eyes, the pleura, lungs, the pericardium, kidneys, connective tissues and the musculature.

There are two forms of this disorder — severe and chronic. In severe cases, there are pain, inflammation and fever. The patient should not perform Yogasans under these circumstances. Asans are beneficial only in a chronic case. It becomes chronic when the disease has been suppressed by the drugs. In a chronic case, there is no inflammation or fever, only pain in the joints.

The reader will be surprised to know that the root-cause of this disorder is digestive disorders, which have occurred earlier in life. The case-history of some patients shows that an attack of constipation and pain in bowels were controlled by drugs. Drugs cure the constipation but the poisonous muck and faeces remain in the intestines. Accumulated poison causes pain and inflammation of the joints.

Garudasan

Garudasan is very beneficial as an exercise of the joints of the arms and legs.

Method: Stand erect, bend the right leg slightly. Curl the left leg on the right leg as if a creeper is going up a tree.

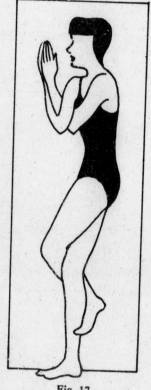

Fig. 17

Bend the upper part of your body slightly forward and curl the arms in the same manner. The two palms should touch each other, after the arms have been curled. This asan is performed while standing on one leg. Beginners may find it difficult. In that case, one can stand against a wall. After the asan has been perfected, there is no need to stand against the wall. Hold the asan as long as you easily can. Inhale and exhale in a peaceful manner and remain relaxed. End the asan and repeat it with left leg curled around the right leg. Interchange the arms too. Repeat four times.

Effect: Garudasan involves movement of joints. This helps the poisonous substances that cause pain to flow out, and the muscles of the joints are exercised. This helps reduce pain. Remember, just performing Garudasan cannot cure the disease. Combine the asans that improve digestion and other treatments.

Badh Padmasan

Sit down on the floor, and stretch the right leg forward. Take hold of the right foot with both hands and,

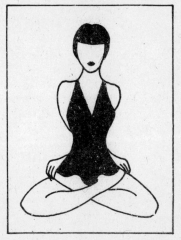

Fig. 18

folding the leg at the knee, place the foot on the left thigh. Similarly, fold the left leg and place it on the right thigh. Keep the body erect and place the hands between the heels one over the other. Keep the breathing normal. This is Padmasan. Now take both arms to the back, place them like a cross, hold the toes of the left foot with the right hand and the toes of the right foot with the left hand. Maintain the asan as long as possible. Increase the duration gradually and with ease. Remember to inhale and exhale normally.

Badh Padmasan has a healthy effect on the joints. The pain in the joints decreases, the digestive system improves, constipation gets cured, the appetite improves, the white glutinous matter stops secreting from the bowels. Chronic patients of rheumatoid arthritis should perform these asans in the following order.

Tanasan — Garudasan — Badh Padmasan — Sarpasan — Shalabhasan — Dhanurasan or Nabhiasan — Pawan Muktasan — Paschimottanasan — Sarvanga.an — Matsyasan — Yogmudra — Shavasan.

DIET REGULATIONS

Food should be nourishing, palatable and adjusted to individual needs and based on personal experience and common sense. A diet high in vitamins and containing adequate protein is advisable. Iron salts may be indicated if iron deficiency or anaemia is present. Avoid cold drinks, radish, curd, buttermilk, rice and some lentils. Do not eat anything that does not agree with your body. Lime juice, mixed with warm water, is very beneficial because sometimes the pain in the joints is caused by acidity in the intestines. Lime is rich in vitamin and this helps improve the vitality of the body and cures constipation. Fomentation can be done in case of excessive pain at any time.

Women's Diseases

All the diseases that have been described in previous chapters are common to men and women. The reproductive organs are the only ones that are not similar in men and women. Therefore the diseases of these organs are referred to as women's diseases affecting the uterus, ovaries and the reproductory organs. The list of diseases connected with these is very long. Modern medical science has written hundreds of volumes about these diseases, and new medicines and treatments have been researched, experimented with and made available.

The major fault with modern medical science, firstly, is that it is spending all its energy on researching and studying an unhealthy body instead of a healthy one. Perhaps it has not been considered necessary to write about the healthy state of the body. Secondly, modern medical science considers most diseases to be localised affairs, whereas a particular disease can be due to general physical debility or to some ailing organ. Long-sightedness is of primary importance. For example, inflammation and collection of uterus or ovaries are caused by constipation and collection of faeces in the intestines. Constipation is caused by lack of exercise and unhealthy food habits. The logical first step should be to cure constipation. The inflamed uterus will cure itself automatically, as the faeces stop affecting it. But if drugs are administered to cure inflammation, they may not create the desired results. Even if the inflammation is reduced to a certain degree, it will recur when the drugs are stopped. I have known a large number of women patients who have suffered from uterus disorders for years, are tired of modern drugs and injections and are still not cured. The reason is lack of far-sightedness. Treatment by Yogasans is particularly beneficial for the diseases of women. Besides the inflammation of the uterus and ovaries, displacement of the uterus, weakness of the uterus and leucorrhea are some of the disorders that are caused by digestive disorders, bad health habits and general debility.

Generally, teenage girls suffer from menstrual disorders. The development of the reproductory organs and their very formation cause menstrual disorders. Whatever the causes, the glands, ovaries and other muscles participating in the menstrual cycle become stiff. Practice of yoga puts pressure on these muscles and glands, blood circulation improves and pure blood is pumped in, which in turn lends strength to the weak and ailing organs.

The same asans as advocated for digestive disorders are beneficial for women's diseases also. The following asans performed in the given order are beneficial for women who have been taking modern drugs for a prolonged period and have not been cured. For the first fifteen days, the order should be as follows:

Tanasan — Garudasan — Badh Padmasan — Pawan Muktasan — Shavasan.

To these, add the following after fifteen days:

Paschimottanasan — Sarpasan — Shalabhasan — Dhanurasan — Nabhiasan — Sarvangasan.

There is no need to include all these at once. Include them gradually. It will depend on an individual's strength. Use your common sense always.

PRECAUTION

Do not perform Yogasans during pregnancy or within the days of menstruation. There are certain asans that can be performed during pregnancy but these must be done under the supervision of a doctor.

The most harmless, easy and effective exercise during pregnancy is a morning walk. This has the same effect as Yogasans. Delivery becomes easy. Yogasans can be started six weeks after delivery.

LOCAL TREATMENT

Fomentation of the parts of the body that lie below the navel, the pubes and the uterus is beneficial for chronic cases. Wet a thick towel with hot water. After fomentation, tie a cloth soaked in cold water (and then squeezed) around the stomach. Tie another woollen scarf or a shawl over this. During summer reduce hot fomentation and replace cold fomentation with a mud bandage.

If this treatment cannot be taken daily, take it at least thrice a week. It cures pain, inflammation and constipation and relieves pain due to menses.

DIET REGULATIONS

Seasonal fruits, raw vegetables, ghee, milk, curd and chapatis made of unsifted flour are beneficial for women who suffer from anaemia, caused by blood loss. Excessive menstrual flow and gastro-intestinal bleeding are the principal causes of blood loss. Normally, Vitamin B 12 and iron capsules are advised. But these do not bring a permanent cure. Raw vegetables and seasonal fruits provide the required iron and vitamins and blood-loss is automatically compensated or made good. The strength of the patient will soon be revive '

Two Important Health Discussions

Uncooked Raw Food

I have indicated the importance of uncooked raw foods in my previous works. But this is a subject that needs a detailed discussion. What I have to say is my personal view-point. A large number of physicians recommend raw food but Ashar Virtar-Hobnneshiah of Teheran (Iran) wrote a book and a pamphlet on the subject and made his theory known to a large number of people. As a result of this, thousands of people the world over have been cured by this system. The writer of this book is a senior official in Iran, practises what he preaches, and his book has been translated into Hindi. He believes that the root-cause of every disease in the world is the eating of cooked food, topped by the consumption of poisonous medicines. He does not consider any medicines given by any system, allopathic, Greek, homoeopathic or ayurvedic, fit for human consumption. He is particularly against modern allopathic drugs because these are manufactured with artificial and unnatural chemicals and are incapable of acting favourably upon the human body. He has called them "fatal poisons." Just like naturopaths, he is against the germ-principle. Raw foods include all those nutritives that are needed by the human body. Cooking food on fire kills all the nutritious substances. Cooked food becomes like garbage for the body. It does not give any nutrition and the body falls victim to disease.

Doctors fail to understand this basic fact. They force poisonous drugs and cooked food into the patient's stomach and turn the body into a junction-point for disease.

The human body has been built up of billions and trillions of cells, tissues and muscles. The live nutritives of uncooked food make the body healthy, give it the power to resist disease. Cooked food can only make the body diseased and sick.

While throwing light on the mysteries and definitions of diseases, he has written that when different parts of the body fail to get complete nutrition, they become hungry for it. The symptoms of various diseases are nothing more than a call from those hungry parts. The need at that time is to deliver the required nutrition to the hungry parts through raw foods. But people do not follow this, undoubtedly as a result of their ignorance. The doctor and the patient repeat their old mistake of taking poisonous drugs and cooked food, which are the main cause of disease, in the first place.

About canned foods and the so called health-giving beverages and tonics, he opines that all these are deceptions, a big mistake and, in fact, nothing but humbug.

The claims that these are nutritious are false, the proteins, vitamins and other minerals that are mixed in these are unnatural. There cannot be a bigger joke cracked at the cost of ailing humanity.

Millions are being spent on research on diseases and germs. Later, more millions are spent on constructing huge laboratories to discover drugs to kill these germs. But what is the result? Diseases keep spreading and increasing in the world, while new drugs keep being discovered, manufactured and consumed.

Modern medicine claims that drugs have conquered a number of diseases and that man is now living longer than before. The truth is that disease is being suppressed by poisonous synthetic medicines, while natural resistance to disease decreases. Consequently, with the passage of time, diseases become chronic. The number of patients suffering from diseases like heart attacks, high blood pressure, asthma, eczema, formation of gas, arthritis and paralysis is on the increase. No medicines can help cure them simply because their bodies are full of the poison of drugs consumed earlier. Cooked food increases the poison every day.

He has included all fruits, uncooked raw vegetables, and sprouted grains, dry fruits, nuts and honey in a balanced diet chart. Milk is not allowed. Any food that has been cooked on fire is not allowed. Those wanting to lead healthy lives should stop eating cooked foods forthwith.

About the difficulties one faces while following this diet regulation, he has written, "A short time after you start on an uncooked raw diet, it is possible that some symptoms of a disease may reappear. But one should not worry and should continue eating raw food only. The body gradually gets used to the changed diet. Never take any other treatment. Wait for the results, which will be encouraging."

He claims that this is the only method that can completely cure any disease, including cancer. Those following these diet regulations never contract any disease, remain healthy, and live for a long time. It is also economical, and one is freed from the tedium of cooking. These diet habits should be inculcated from childhood. To give cooked food to children is to cheat them of a healthy life.

THE PRINCIPLE OF UNCOOKED FOOD

There is absolutely no doubt that uncooked food is

very nutritious. There is ample proof that this system is helpful in curing diseases. Thousands of people who have become disease-free through this system will vouch for its effectiveness.

The thesis that modern drugs are poisonous for the human body is valid. These drugs give birth to new diseases and possibly revive old maladies. Naturopaths are in agreement with this system. The only difference is that in naturopathy the help of water, mud bandages and regulated food is taken, while this system is against any kind of treatment. They believe that raw uncooked food is the master-key for curing all ailments.

The only thing I find objectionable in this system is its rigidity. It is unscientific to run after any principle with a closed mind. No scientist ever believes that any achievement of his is complete or unchangeable. New research always shows a new way. Old beliefs and principles have to be changed or discarded. There are some arguments against the consumption of uncooked, that is, raw food. Why did man start cooking food on fire? Where and when did he acquire the knowledge of cooking?

One story is that when early man lived in jungles, he ate mainly meat. One day, they say, the jungle caught fire. Next morning the people found some birds which had been literally roasted alive in the fire. They were forced to eat the birds in order to satisfy their pangs of hunger. Everyone liked the roasted meat and found that it was digested more easily and more quickly. Man then invented fire. Whether that is actually how man started roasting and cooking his food, the fact remains that over thousands of years past, man's digestive system has got used to cooked food.

That cooked food is the root-cause of disease is no longer hundred per cent true, since man's digestive system has got used to cooked food. There are thousands of people who eat normal cooked food and do not contract any disease for very long periods of time. They must be following some other health regulations.

All those who lived up to a hundred years or more were used to cooked food. There must be a secret of their longevity.

Food cooked on fire is easily digestible, while uncooked food, particularly sprouted grains, is hard to digest. Often sprouted grains can be detected whole in the bowels. These were obviously not digested, although that could be due to ineffective or incomplete digestion.

It is difficult to decide what kind of uncooked food should be eaten and in what quantity.

The kind of society we are living in today is not very sympathetic to anyone wanting to eat uncooked food. Eating raw food in today's world is as problematic as a vegetarian looking for food in a predominantly non-vegetarian country. If a person is used to raw, uncooked food and if he is someone's guest, both he and the host face difficulties. Those eating uncooked food are often deprived of the enjoyment of sitting with friends and eating with them.

Besides these practical difficulties, there is also the possibility of certain other problems that may prove to be health hazards.

A reader of my books has written to me, "I have been a patient of nervous break-down for the past eight years. I started eating uncooked food from 12th June 1976 onwards. My diet included sprouted grains, vegetables, seasonal fruits and honey. Within five months, I was completely cured. I have been living on uncooked food for the past eleven months. But I have become very weak. I even find it hard to move around. According to the book that I used as a guide for my treatment, this weakness is a matter for cleansing. When cleansing is complete, strength returns automatically. Are you in agreement with this theory? I need directions. I wrote two letters to Iran. They sent some publicity material and photographs. I am very upset and cannot decide what I should do. Can you guide me? I shall be very grateful if you can help me."

The problem was not one of cleansing. He was not getting any carbohydrates and fats from the uncooked food. These two substances give energy and strength to our body. Therefore the raw food that he was eating did not constitute a balanced diet, which must include the following:

1. Proteins: Proteins are the main constituents of the body. Just as a machine undergoes wear and tear when it is used, similarly our body also undergoes wear and tear and can be repaired only by proteins provided by food. For vegetarians three proteins are available in the form of sprouted lentils and dry fruits and nuts. Milk, eggs and meat have proteins in plenty. However, they are all banned for those eating uncooked raw food.

2. Mineral salts: For the growth and restoration of the body, minerals are the next most important substance. The body contains twenty minerals, all of which must be replenished from food. 1/25th part of the body consists of different minerals. Minerals are needed for bone formation. Like proteins, minerals are also a protective food of high biological value, and have to be replaced through food. All foods contain one or another mineral. But raw vegetables and fruits are the richest in minerals. Lack of these minerals can cause rickets, tetany, hyper-irritability, decay of teeth, and excessive bleeding due to delayed coagulation. Lack of iodine can cause goitre and an enlargement of the thyroid glands.

3. Carbohydrates: Carbohydrates serve as the main source of energy to the body. When consumed in excess, they may be converted into fat and stored in the body. The carbohydrates present in foodstuffs include starch and various sugars. Starch is contained in white flour, rice, sago, starchy foods. Sugar is found in sugar, jaggery, honey, unrefined sugar, etc.

These carbohydrates have only one function — they serve as a source of energy. Those doing hard physical labour need more carbohydrates. Those doing less physical work need less carbohydrates.

4. Fats: Fats serve as a source of energy along with carbohydrates, and are also stored in the body beneath the skin and, to some extent, in other parts. Fat in the diet serves as a carrier for the fat-soluble vitamins A, D, E and K. Fat also supplies certain essential fatty acids which are needed by the body.

5. Vitamins: A lot is said about vitamins these days. Apart from proteins, carbohydrates, fats and minerals, there are certain other substances present in minute quantities in most foodstuffs and are necessary for proper growth and health. These are called vitamins. Several vitamins have been isolated so far, but for human beings, the most important are vitamin A and carotene, vitamin D, vitamin B and riboflavin, vitamin C, vitamin B12, folic acid.

A large continued deficiency of these vitamins causes a number of disorders, which are called deficiency diseases. Deficiency of vitamin C, for example, causes the disease known as scurvy. This disease is characterised by weakness and irritability, bleeding under the skin, pain in the joints, swelling and bleeding of gums, anaemia. It can also cause weakening of the bones, which then fracture easily. Raw vegetables and seasonal fruits are the best source for all vitamins. Uncooked raw foods provide these in plenty. That most vitamins are destroyed while cooking, frying, and roasting is a self-evident proposition and a widely known fact now.

Refer now to the reader whose letter I have reproduced earlier. By living on raw food for eleven months, he recovered from his disease. But he became very weak. I have already mentioned that his diet was not balanced. He was not getting sufficient fat or carbohydrates from the uncooked food. The main sources of fat and carbohydrates are not permitted in this system.

I have also mentioned that this system is too rigid. If

my young reader had made adequate changes in his diet, he could have maintained his energy and strength. I shall repeat once again, understand the principle, the scientific point of view, and then take a line of treatment. He should have included milk, curd, ghee and jaggery in his diet. It is erroneous to think that these foods can cause some other disease.

The principle of a balanced diet applies equally to cooked and uncooked food. The meaning of a balanced diet is only this that all the five substances should be present in the food in the required quantities. Each human being is a separate individualistic entity in himself. The requirements of food intake depend upon age, height, weight, sex, physical activity and the nature of work done by each human being. Dieticians have prepared detailed tables for different kinds of lifestyle.

Much has been written about food. But is it possible or practical for an ordinary person to measure the food he eats every day?

Animals in the jungle do not measure their food. They use their common sense. New-born babies have lots of common sense. They do not drink milk if they are not hungry. Gradually, as a human being grows, he starts losing this common sense. On certain occasions, without any conscious provocation, our common sense is awakened. Suddenly we want to eat a guava or some other thing. One must eat that thing. That particular food is beneficial for health. On this, perhaps, is based the saying "Jo ruche so pache" (that which is palatable is also digestible).

WHAT TO DO

After reading so much about cooked and uncooked food, readers must be wanting to know how to benefit from uncooked food and how to remove the practical difficulties mentioned above.

In my opinion, if people suffering from a stubborn

chronic disease follow the programme of curing themselves with uncooked food, they will certainly benefit, provided they follow the regulations strictly. I am against switching to uncooked food suddenly. Start with plenty of raw vegetables and seasonal fruits. Eat these at one meal and boiled vegetables and two wheat chapatis for the second meal. After a couple of days, stop eating chapatis and continue eating boiled vegetables. And then start eating sprouted grains. Moong is the lightest of all foodgrains. It is advisable to start with whole sprouted moong. Later add wheat, peanuts, soyabeans, etc. and gradually start eating only uncooked food. But remember the following:

1. Young people seldom have any disorder due to eating uncooked food because their body is strong and healthy. Older people may encounter some problems as they are not so able-bodied and strong.

2. If the disease is aggravated or if, during the act of cleansing, any physical discomfort is experienced, go on a fast or use the mud and water method of naturopathy. Curd, milk, ghee, unrefined sugar and jaggery should be taken if one feels weak. Dry fruits and nuts like almonds, cashewnuts, walnuts, kismish, pistas, etc. are included in the uncooked, raw-food diet table. But these are very expensive. So one can include coconuts, dates and walnuts in plenty. One should not hesitate to eat roasted peanuts. You must use your commonsense and make the necessary changes according to your body's requirements.

DIET TABLE FOR GOOD HEALTH

Only those suffering from a stubborn chronic disease are attracted to the system of treatment by an uncooked, raw diet. No one turns to this system merely for good health. In fact, there is no need for this. If a person, keen on maintaining good health, decides on a diet with thought and care, he can keep healthy all his life. What should the diet table be? What kind of food should be taken? First I would like to introduce my readers to some facts connected with the preparation of food.

All seasonal fruits, raw vegetables and sprouted grains are very beneficial and strength-giving. The body receives all the nutritive substances through these.

Roasted corn, peanuts, cashewnuts, soyabeans, etc., are second on the table of nutritive foods. Very little of the nutritive substances is lost during roasting and such foods are easy to digest. Similarly, chapatis cooked on low fire and lightly boiled vegetables lose very little of their nutritive value. Food cooked on low fire is also easy to digest. Prolonged cooking destroys all the nutritives just as fried foods lose all the nutritive substances. Such foods should never be eaten.

Based on these facts, a mixed food diet regulation is suitable for good health and a disease-free life. What kind of diet table should a person make? It will depend entirely on that person's taste, lifestyle, social and economic position. The choice of the diet table will be different for each country and time.

UNCOOKED, COOKED, MIXED FOOD

In North India, parathas and puris are stuffed with ground urad dal. Samosas sold in the market are stuffed with uncooked peas and cauliflower. But because these are fried, their nutritive value is considerably reduced.

It is very beneficial to grate raw radish, carrots, marrow or chopped fenugreek leaves, or spinach and make stuffed chapatis or parathas. Chapatis should not be over-cooked. The nutritive substances of the stuffed vegetables remain intact, the vegetables become soft and are easy to eat. This kind of mixed uncooked-cooked food is very delicious, nutritive and easy to digest.

The Search for Sanjivani Plant

A very popular episode from the *Ramayana* is the battle between Rama and Ravana. Meghnad shot a *Shakti Baan* at Laxmana. Consequently, Laxmana fainted. It was not an ordinary unconsciousness. A Vaid was called from Lanka who said that Laxmana could only be revived by the Sanjivani plant. This was available only on the Gandhi-Madan Mountain. Hanuman, after a lot of effort, went and brought the Sanjivani plant which revived Laxmana. Since then Sanjivani plant is considered to be the symbol of treatment for all diseases. No one knows where it grows and whether actually it exists or not. But physicians of the world are searching for a herb or a plant that can cure all diseases and promote the health of humanity.

Wheat Grass

In the recent past, much has been said about wheat grass and its juice. Many journalists published articles on how to use it. It became famous and was compared to the Sanjivani plant. Many public institutions and some generous people published material giving information about it and distributed it free. But these publications and booklets gave very limited information. A vast number of doubts remained. The information given by Lt. Col (retired) Satanandji in his journal "Iron Federation" is detailed and complete. Here are some excerpts.

The research in this field has been done by an American doctor, N. Wigmore. Dr. Wigmore wrote a book called *Amrit Tulya Gehun ki Ghas*. Wigmore believes that theoretically man can live a healthy life till the age of a thousand years.

According to the Bible, the earth consists of 103 chemical substances and grass is the only substance that contains all these chemicals. Grass is the special diet of animals and man is a special animal.

94

After years of research on 4700 kinds of grass, it has been proved that wheat grass is the king of all grasses. Its juice contains the maximum number of nutritive substances. It has been administered to thousands of patients who had been declared incurable.

The grass specialist, **Dr. Yarp** Thomas, wrote in 1962, "Grass contains chlorophyl. This is the richest nutritive substance." Dr. Thomas has been researching and working on the grasses for more than fifty years.

Dr. Wigmore has cured patients who had been given up by physicians, simply by making them drink three glasses of wheat grass juice every day. Their diet consisted of simple boiled vegetables and fruits. Some of the examples of these cures are:

1. An old man, whose waist was completely bent, was cured.

2. A patient of wind, whose knees and ankles were inflammed, was cured within three weeks.

3. A seventy-year-old woman had been suffering from boils in the intestines. The boils on her body had pus. She was cured within a month.

4. A bishop in Syria lost his voice. For years, he suffered due to various other diseases and became very weak. He benefited from wheat grass so much that he started performing his duties like a young man.

5. Even a patient of leprosy drank three glasses of fresh wheat grass juice and was cured after a year.

5. For 14 years, a 65-year-old patient of throat cancer took treatment from at least a hundred institutions and doctors. Dr. Wigmore started administering a large glass of wheat grass juice every two hours four times a day. Within five days, the foul odour stopped. Fomentation was done with wheat grass. Within two weeks, pus formation stopped. He got his voice back within a fortnight and wounds in the throat were cured, and the holes were sealed. He was completely cured within two

months. Plastic surgery was performed on his face and he became healthy and handsome once again.

7. Another cancer patient was cured within 6 months with this treatment.

8. At least 10,000 patients have written to Dr. Wigmore after being cured by his treatment.

A large number of kidney and diabetic patients have been cured. Even loss of hair and greying can be stopped. Fomentation with wheat grass helps relieve headaches, constipation, boils, piles and burns. Alcoholics have also been cured by this.

You do not need a doctor for this treatment. You can grow your own wheat at home and treat yourself. Within three weeks, it will make you fresh, youthful and healthy.

How to Grow Wheat Grass

1. Take a number of 8-inch-deep, 20-inch-wide and 30-inch-long boxes. Fill them with ordinary manure and good earth.

2. Soak wheat (it should be free of fertiliser manure) at night, sprinkle the wheat in the boxes in the morning. Spread half an inch layer of earth.

3. Water the boxes well till the wheat is set. Reduce the quantity of water after the seeds have sprouted. Within seven days of sprouting the wheat-grass will be ready for use. Space out the seed sowing, so that you can have fresh grass every day.

4. When the grass is five to seven inches long, cut it, wash it and then grind it and extract juice. You can add ground mint leaves and honey to the juice. *Never add salt, fruit juice, vegetable extract or lime to wheat grass juice.* These should be consumed separately.

5. Wheat grass can be grown in any season. The boxes should be placed in a shady place. Direct sunlight should not fall on the plants.

6. After cutting the grass, remove the roots from the box. Sow fresh wheat in its place.

7. It is beneficial to eat boiled vegetables and fruits. Goat's or cow's milk and an occasional fast are also beneficial.

8. Some people start vomiting and get an attack of diarrhoea. There is no need to panic. Vomiting and loose motions will stop automatically.

9. Wheat grass can be sprinkled on vegetables or added to wheat flour chapatis just like coriander leaves.

SPECIAL PRECAUTIONS ABOUT GRASS JUICE

The juice must be consumed within three hours of extraction. Its effect is lost if kept for too long. Do not gulp the juice quickly, sip it slowly. Dose: In a healthy state, drink three to four ounces at a time. Upto 200 or 250 grams should be taken at a time if sick. (Courtesy: Shri Satanand, Editor, "Iron Federation".)

A NATURAL DOUBT

Can every disease be cured by the juice of the wheat grass? This question has been asked by many.

It can cure all diseases but it is not certain that all patients can be cured. It all depends on the vitality of the patient. No doubt the chlorophyl in this grass gives strength and vitality to a patient. But this is as true as that fire can only be lighted if there is a spark and fuel. Without a spark, you cannot light a fire, no matter how much coal or firewood you have.

Similarly, if you do not have the strength to digest wheat grass juice and render it beneficial to the body, the question of curing the patient does not arise. Even the other methods of naturopathy demand vitality and strength. Any patient whose vitality is low cannot be saved.

REACTION TO TREATMENT

There is no question of any ill-effects or after-effects

of wheat grass juice because it is not prepared in laboratories with artificial chemicals. It contains natural substances which match very well with the human body. The vomiting or loose motions mentioned above are only part of the process of cleansing. Vomiting and loose motions only help the poisons of the body to be thrown out. Although this need not happen to everyone, it speeds up the treatment.

PROCESS OF BECOMING HEALTHY

As already mentioned in the last chapter, the first requirement of a healthy body is protein. Those drinking wheat grass juice do not have to eat meat nor do they have to drink milk. The required quantity of proteins is available in this. It is rich not only in protein but also in minerals and vitamins. One of its contents, chlorophyll, is also called "green blood". Dr. Wigmore claims that if a person eats a spoonful of wheat grass every day, all his needs of dietary substances are fulfiled.

For good health, wheat grass and its juice are very beneficial. While it cures all diseases, it provides the best tonic too.

There is no doubt that if wheat grass is consumed every day, one can be cured of all ailments. One can lead a healthy, happy life. Some find the whole exercise very laborious and troublesome. But for extraordinary gains, extraordinary labour has to be put in.

Appendix

HIP-BATH

The father of treatment with water in the naturopathic system, Louikuhe, discovered a variety of baths. Hip-bath is an effective and special bath in his system. As the name indicates, this bath involves the stomach and hips. This bath is taken in a special kind of tub. This is not a usual round tub. One part of the tub has a back rest. Such tubs are available easily.

Fill fresh water in a tub from a well or a handpump. Fill up enough water so that when you sit in the tub, the water should be a little above your navel. Undress and sit down in the tub. The legs should be outside the tub, place the legs on a stool, place a pillow behind your back. Take a small soft towel or a muslin cloth. Put it on the abdomen and rub from right to left and then from left to right. Repeat three or four times. Rub the area near the navel. In the beginning, take the hip-bath for 10 minutes, increase the duration to 30 minutes gradually. After the hip-bath, come out, wipe the body and wear light clothing.

Special: Asthma patients should use warm water. They should take the hip-bath in a closed room.

MUD BANDAGE

Mud is a major element of treatment in naturopathy. Father Nipe and Adolf Joost, the leading doyens of naturopathy, have stressed the effectiveness and use of mud. It is natural that our body, which already has a large portion of earth in it, should benefit by this. Besides, it is available everywhere. Earth has a lot of strength that pulls out the poisons and heat from diseases.

The earth near rivers and streams is very beneficial. But if this is not available, take mud from a clean place. Never take mud from a farm or from places used by people for defecating. Dig at least one metre deep before taking the mud. Before soaking the mud, remove all grass, straws, pebbles and clean it. Mix enough water and make it into a thick dough. Mud cakes for eyes need less water.

MUD BANDAGE FOR ABDOMEN

Spread mud on a cloth long and wide enough to go around the abdomen. The layer of the mud dough should be half an inch thick. If it is feared that the bandage will fall, tie another bandage over the mud bandage. It should remain tied to the abdomen for at least one hour. If applied at night, let it remain tied for the entire night.

ENEMA

The aim of enema is to cleanse the stomach. A variety of enema containers are available. But the best is the one made of enamelware.

It is easy to take an enema. Hang the tank of the container on the wall. The containers are available in a variety of sizes. The most suitable is the three-pint one. On the outer side is fixed a two-inch-long tube, to this is attached another tube made of rubber or plastic. At the end of the tube is fixed a spout for drawing water. To the front part of this spout is fixed the enema nozzle. It is the nozzle that is inserted in the rectum.

Method: Lie down straight or on your left side. The enema tank should be one metre above the bed. Beginners should not use more than two kilos of water.

Use lukewarm water, if constipated. Do not add anything to the water except the juice of one lime. Before inserting the nozzle, remove a little water by opening the spout, so that water is not blocked. Apply a little oil or vaseline on the nozzle for easy insertion. The nozzle should be cleaned well before and after use.

Basically, the water should be retained in the body for as long as possible, so that the passage of faeces is complete. It takes time to learn retention of water. Turn over in the bed a couple of times. Pat the stomach lightly. Evacuate bowels only when fully pressurised.

Bowel movement after an enema is preceded by passing of whitish liquid, followed by dirty liquid and faeces and finally solid excrement.

Never rush or pressurise evacuation of bowel. It is advisable to sit for 20 or even 30 minutes in the bathroom. Sometimes one feels that some liquid has been retained in the stomach. Do not worry about it. It goes out by itself after some time.

For deriving benefit from the enema, drink half a kilo of water 15 minutes before taking an enema.

One can take a bath immediately after an enema. But do not take an enema immediately after a meal.

Glossary

English	Hindi
Acacia	Keekar
Almonds	Badam
Alum water	Fitkari ka pani
Aniseed	Saunf
Asafoetida	Hing
Ayurvedic preparation	"Lavan Bhaskar Chooran"
Basil leaf	Tulsi
Betel leaf	Paan
Bitter gourd	Karela
Black gram	Kala channa
Black pepper	Kali mirch
Black plum	Jamun
Black salt	Kala namak
Buttermilk	Lassi
Calcium carbonate	Chuna
Caraway seeds	Shahzeera
Cardamoms	Elaichi
Cashewnuts	Kaju
Catechu	Katha
Cinnamon	Dalchini
Cloves	Lavang
Coconut	Narial
Cumin seeds	Zeera
Curd (Yoghurt)	Dahi
Dried grapes	Munakkas
Fenugreek	Methi
Fig flowers	Anjeer ke phool
Flour	Maida
Ginger	Adrak
Green gram	Moong dal
Guavas	Amrud
Honey	Shehad, madhu

English	Hindi
Jaggery	Gur
Lime (Lemon)	Nimboo
Linseed	Alsi
Margosa tree	Neem tree
Marrow	Ghia
Mint leaves	Pudina
Mulberry leaves	Shatoot ke patte
Muskmelon	Kharbooza
Muslin	Mulmul
Myrobalan	Amla
Myrobalan preserved in sugar syrup	Amla murabba
Peanuts	Moongphalli
Pipal	Pipal
Pistachios	Pista
Raisins	Kishmish
Rice and milk pudding	Kheer
Rice husk	Isabgol
Ridge gourd	Torai
Roasted Corn	Makka
Sago	Sagodana
Sal ammoniac	Nosadar
Soda-bi-carb	Soda
Spinach	Palak
Sugarcane juice	Ganne ka ras
Sugar crystals	Mishri
Turnip	Shalgum
Unrefined sugar	Shakkar
Walnuts	Akhrot
Watermelon	Tarbooz
Wheat grass	Gehun ghas
Wheat husk	Gehun ka chhilka or bhussi
White sugar	Cheeni
Wood apple	Bael

DR. LAKSHMINARAIN SHARMA

YOGA

◆ for the cure of ◆

COMMONDISEASES

Yoga for the Cure of Common Diseases is a handy guide to radiant health the natural way without medication.

Written by a famous doctor for the benefit of every home, this authoritative book will assist you to maintain the health of your family through yogasanas. These asanas are simple to perform and produce near miraculous results. They provide remedies for curing many common diseases.

The yogasanas which take only a few minutes a day will help you prolong the span of your life. By following this unique yoga plan, you will be able to lead a long and healthy life.

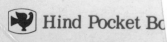 Hind Pocket Bo

8121600138

Rs. 25